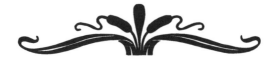

Raw Power!

Building Strength and Muscle Naturally

Stephen Arlin
www.rawfood.com

**Published by
Maul Brothers Publishing
San Diego, California**

Raw Power!
by Stephen Arlin

Disclaimer:
This book is not intended as medical advice because Mr. Arlin does not recommend the use of cooked foods or medicines to alleviate health challenges. Because there is always some risk involved, the author, publisher, and/or distributors of this book are not responsible for any adverse consequences or detoxification effects resulting from the use of any procedures or dietary suggestions described hereafter. Simply put, you are responsible for yourself!

First Edition: August 1, 1998
Third Edition: September 1, 2002
Cover Art: Ken Seaney, Ground Zero Graphic Design
ISBN #0-9653533-5-4

Printed in North America by
Maul Brothers Publishing
PO Box 900202
San Diego, CA 92190 USA
(619) 645-7282

For a FREE catalog, call (888) RAW-FOOD
or visit www.rawfood.com

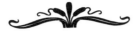

Acknowledgments

This book is dedicated to the truth and health seekers of the world.

I would like to thank my mother Susan, my business partner and lifelong friend David Wolfe, and the amazing Nature's First Law staff.

Special thanks to my wife Jolie and my sons William and Schön, who are my raison d'etre. Thanks to Jolie for her support and all of her work on this book; thanks to our boys for teaching us both so much.

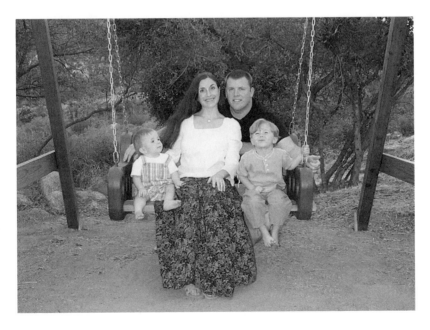

Schön, Jolie, Stephen, and Will at home in California.

Also by Stephen Arlin:

Nature's First Law: The Raw-Food Diet (book)

How to Win an Argument With a
Cooked-Food Eater (audio tape)

Major Achievements of the
Cooked Food Eater (booklet)

IS Philosophy (manifesto)

Available through:
Nature's First Law
PO Box 900202
San Diego, CA 92190 U.S.A.
(619) 645-7282
(800) 205-2350 - orders only
http://www.rawfood.com
nature@rawfood.com

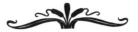

Table of Contents

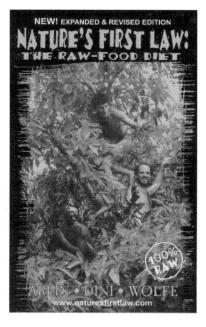

www.rawfood.com

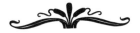

Introduction

Back in 1994, I remember thinking, "If The Raw-Food Diet cures so-called 'incurable' illnesses and rejuvenates old, tired, and diseased bodies, what would happen if someone who was relatively healthy adopted The Raw-Food Diet?" Well, that thought led me and my organization to one of the greatest discoveries in the history of the world—Paradise Health. Our San Diego, California-based organization is Nature's First Law. We have written a controversial raw-foods book entitled **Nature's First Law: The Raw-Food Diet** and we are out there every day delivering this vital message to the world.

It was the reading and self-education we did on health, disease, and diet that led us to The Raw-Food Diet. We focused only on success—success stories, people who had healed themselves of disease, people who lived the longest and healthiest, people who had traveled and observed human beings all over the world. We did not focus on the standard medical dogma as that has largely been a failure. (There is more disease, sickness, and misery now than ever before in human history.) We started bouncing ideas off of each other and we really got into some amazing things.

It was challenging at first because cooked food is addictive and getting over any addiction is tough—but worth it! For every disciplined effort in life there is a multiple reward. Once I cleansed my body of the cooked-food residues, I no longer craved cooked food. What a liberating experience! I can sincerely tell you it is magical. When I went all-raw, I opened up the natural part of my consciousness that had been locked up in a dark dungeon all my life. I see the world more clearly now.

Every day is a great day. All my desires become realized much more quickly now. It may sound strange, but it is true.

As soon as I realized that eating cooked food was unnatural and that it was the cause of many human health problems, I took massive raw-foods action. I just did my best each day to go without cooked food and I didn't worry about how much raw plant food I was eating. There is a saying: "Every amount of raw plant food is better than any amount of cooked food." I used to eat a lot of raw food back then, but that subsided as soon as I got over my cooked-food addiction. I stopped eating cooked food completely after about a year.

The level of health I have attained is indescribable, incomprehensible, and unfathomable to people who haven't experienced 100% raw-foodism. It's the difference between night and day. It's the difference between an inner-city slum and a tropical paradise. I shed 51 unwanted, unhealthy pounds (238 to 187—I'm 6'2") and have since then gained back 40 pounds of healthy, solid muscle through the unique training work-outs and 100% raw-plant-food diet outlined in this book.

I currently eat (by weight) about 60% raw, organic fruit, 30% raw, organic, green-leafy vegetables, and 10% raw, organic nuts and sunflower seeds. Note that I'm using the botanical definition of fruit: a fruit is something that contains the seeds within itself for regeneration of the plant. (Avocado, olive, tomato, cucumber, squash, pepper, etc. are all botanically fruits.)

This diet is easy, once you know the facts. No one could have the discipline to do this diet if there wasn't something going on biologically. Eating cooked food has nothing to do with the normal biological requirements of the cells. Food put to flame becomes addictive. Once you break away from that you open yourself up to a most incredible personal discovery.

Today's heresy is tomorrow's orthodoxy. Nature's First Law represents a force of resistance against enormous odds. We are at the forefront of a movement which proposes to reshape the world. Therefore, we serve the future and not just the passing hour. The greatest and most enduring successes in history are those which were least understood in the beginning, because they were in strong contrast to public opinion and the majority views and wishes of the time. Every great idea once began on the fringe.

There is a lot of conflicting information in the world today, especially in the field of nutrition. However, there is one thing that is certain: every living organism on Planet Earth is designed to nourish themselves with raw nutrition, and humans are certainly no exception. A raw-foodist is not something you become, it is something you already are. Every single natural organism on the planet eats exclusively raw foods. No free-living creature ever tampers with its food. Some people consider this diet the next step past a vegetarian or vegan diet, but it really transcends all diets. It is simply the natural way to nourish your body.

This book is about attaining a level of health that is our absolute birthright—Paradise Health. It is about eating a 100% *natural* diet, *true* natural body-building, and *total* fitness. What is known to the world as "Natural Body-Building" is hardly natural at all. Just because someone trains steroid-free, it doesn't mean they are building a natural body. Food is the foundation of everything we are physically. If you are eating unnatural food, you are engaged in "Unnatural Body-Building." The only way to truly build your body is through eating naturally. This book does not spend much time presenting arguments in favor of The Raw-Food Diet. It assumes that the reader already has a basic knowledge of what true natural nutrition is—raw food. If you do in fact want a comprehensive overview of the entire philosophy of natural raw-food nutrition, I recommend first reading **Nature's First Law: The Raw-Food Diet** by Arlin, Dini, and Wolfe.

The Information Age, in many ways, has become overbearing and obsolete. Listening to and acting upon your own body's natural instincts, desires, and needs is the way to Paradise Health, not by listening to someone else's dietary dogma.

Best wishes,
Stephen Arlin

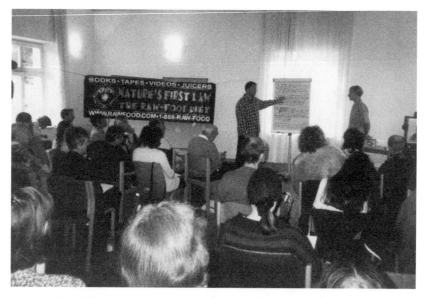

Stephen presents his "Raw Power! Seminar"
just outside of Munich, Germany during the
Nature's First Law 2000 European Tour.

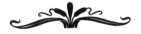

Raw Power!

Conversations between healers and patients through the ages.
PATIENT: I have a headache.
HEALER: 2000 B.C. - Here, eat this fruit.
1000 A.D. - That fruit is heathen, say this prayer.
1850 A.D. - That prayer is superstition, drink this potion.
1940 A.D. - That potion is snake oil, swallow this pill.
1985 A.D. - That pill is ineffective, take this antibiotic.
2000 A.D. - That antibiotic is artificial. Here, eat this fruit.

Every living organism on Planet Earth is naturally a 100% raw-food eater; not 99%, not 70%, not 50%—100%! There are trillions of organisms and creatures on this planet that are thriving and living virtually disease-free eating 100% raw foods. There is only one organism that tampers with its food—the human organism. *Trillions to one!* Those are staggering odds. That would make the likelihood that we should be eating cooked food about 100,000 times more improbable than winning the lottery. You don't want to bet against those kind of odds. Eat all raw!

I know raw-foodists all over the world, in just about every country. I have met raw-foodists that live in inner cities; I have met raw-foodists that live in tropical paradises. The point is, no matter where you live, no matter what condition you live in, you can make the change and eat 100% raw foods—every living organism on this planet does it, and so can you.

Most health-seekers give up on the raw-food diet when their weight drops and the peer criticism and self-doubt begins.

This book is designed to help you reach the next level, to surpass the negativity, and to build a body filled with super-strength and energy!

When you first adopt The Raw-Food Diet you will lose weight. It is inevitable. After years of eating cooked and processed dead foods, your body becomes loaded with toxic material. For example, the only way to clean a bathtub filled with dirty water is to pull out the plug and let it completely drain. Once the body has a chance to unload poisons, it will do so. Each organ will cleanse itself, every tissue will purge dead material. The body will detoxify. This is always accompanied by weight loss. "The good will push out the bad."

This detoxification process is the major barrier to achieving a 100% raw-food diet, especially if you are advanced in years. Cooked food clogs up your body and stops detoxification, so to properly detoxify, you must combat cooked-food addiction. Get the cooked food out, bring the raw food in! How do you clean up the river as long as the chemical plant is dumping waste into it?

Do you remember the concept of diffusion from chemistry class? Molecules move from areas of greater concentration to areas of lesser concentration. As the blood thins out on The Raw-Food Diet, toxic, undigested molecules trapped in the lymph will pour into the blood.

As one keeps rinsing, washing, and polishing the membranous tract, one may experience recurring symptoms of past illnesses. Coughs, colds, headaches, mucus eliminations, diarrhea, sore throats, fevers, rashes, pains that float from one part of the body to another, and the negative mental states of anxiety, depression, and imbalance, may reappear as one persists with a natural lifestyle of raw foods, exercise, and sunshine. Your weight will fall.

To win through, you must endure all these discomforts, even if you have to relive (for short periods of time) old sicknesses experienced as far back as your childhood. The toxins and wastes responsible for old sicknesses, which may have lain dormant since infancy, will be released from their hiding places. You may even taste a medicine you ingested years back, or have a craving for a food you have not eaten in decades. I have suddenly tasted breakfast cereals not eaten in fifteen years.

The cycles of purge and replenishment may last weeks, months, or even a couple of years. It all depends on your lifestyle before. It depends on how toxic your body is. Everybody goes through a different detoxification process. *Embrace the detoxification process, accept it, and get past it.*

During the detoxification period and the initial stages of raw eating, you can and should, exercise the muscles and strengthen the body. While exercising, you may experience light-headedness and other detoxification symptoms. You may not feel as strong, because your body is using all of its energy to cleanse and rebuild itself. Always do what you can, where you are, with what you have. Start walking and build up from there if that's what it takes.

You will not put on healthy weight until the body is sufficiently cleansed. Again, this may take a couple of months for some people or a couple of years for others, depending on their age and the toxic conditions of their bodies. In my case, I lost 51 pounds (23 kg) initially. I dropped from 238 pounds (107 kg) to 187 pounds (84 kg) and stayed at that weight for 4-5 months when I was transitioning. Then I quickly gained 15 pounds back (6.8 kg) (by exercising and eating the exact same raw food diet) and have steadily been gaining weight ever since. Now, I weigh approximately 225 pounds (102 kg)—I'm 6'2" tall.

Anyone can gain all the strength and healthy weight they want, in any parts of their bodies they choose. Whether you want to gain 10, 20, or 30 pounds (4.5, 9, 13.5 kg), you can! If you gain just one wholesome pound per month, in one year, you will gain 12 pounds (5.5 kg)! Remember, your bodyweight is 50% muscle.

Look at every part of your body in the mirror, daily. Look for challenging areas. Exercise where you need development. The areas of your body you consider to be thin or underweight are the areas upon which you should focus your attention and energy.

On The Raw-Food Diet, it is easy to gain muscle and unleash a hidden strength and potential if you will persist past the negativity and peer pressure. No great success is possible without persistence. Change your peer group if necessary. Get away from toxic people. Water seeks its own level, and you can rest assured that people will try to bring you down to their level.

It's definitely not an overnight transformation, although you can start to see results immediately. You obviously can't expect to be in perfect physical shape by working-out once. The same is true with anything for that matter. Fundamentals practiced daily and consistently produce massive results.

To gain healthy, muscular weight, you must do all you can of the following:

1. think powerfully!
2. eliminate artificial substances, drugs and medicines
3. engage in intense resistance exercises
4. sunbathe (nude if possible)
5. maintain your emotional poise
6. be free of toxic environments
7. only consume liquids when ill
8. get adequate sleep
9. meditate
10. avoid sexual overindulgence

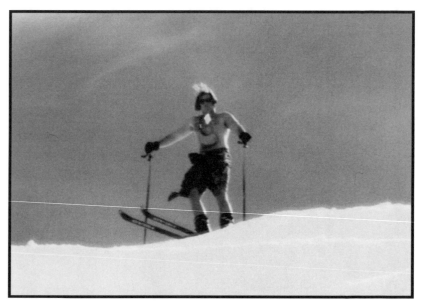

Since adopting The Raw-Food Diet several years ago, I have experienced a major increase in my body's resistance to extreme weather temperatures. I am much more resistant to cold and hot weather now than I was before. Snow-skiing without a shirt (or clothes) feels great!

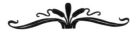

Power of the Mind

If you have the belief that you can do it,
you shall surely acquire the capacity to do it,
even if you do not have it at the beginning.

Human potential is unlimited. There is no point where your memory is too good, your creativity too high, your thought process too clear, your intuition too strong, or your extra sensory too powerful—there is no ceiling! The human mind is truly amazing.

The most important factor in attaining the exact physique that you desire is mind, or attitude. Have you heard of the "Self-Fulfilling Prophecy?" If you truly believe something, it is more likely to come true. If you truly make a concerted effort to gain muscle and healthy weight, you can do it. You must conclusively decide that you *want* to gain strength and weight and make it your number one priority. Write down your goal weight and physique on paper (in your journal). To achieve your goal, a vision of the peak is needed, for the first step depends on the last. Imagine or picture your body as it will look when you achieve your goal physique.

When the going gets tough, it is always the mind that fails first, not the body. What you think about comes about. Closely monitor the conversation and pictures you allow to fill your mind.

Affirm in your own mind, "I am strong; I am powerful; I am unstoppable; I can gain strength and healthy weight each day." Look at yourself in the mirror and emotionally tell your-self "You cannot be stopped; You are energized; You are unlim-ited." This is the mindset of a winner. Do you think Olympic athletes beat themselves up daily with their own thoughts? No way! Winners first become winners in their minds. They affirm their own capabilities daily, either in their conscious mind, out loud, on paper, or all three. You must do the same. As long as you are thinking "I am weak," you will be weak. Weak thoughts lead one to progressively identify with weak-ness. Challenge yourself, use your mind to strengthen your determination, strength, and resolve. Do it, never doubt it. One doubt, and you're out. If at first you don't succeed, try again! Life is a roller coaster, not a merry-go-round. Hang in there!

The notion that incredible strength and healthy weight cannot be built on a raw-food, vegetarian regime is simply that... a notion. A notion that has absolutely no basis in fact. The 200-pound (91-kg) body of the orangutan, the 500-pound (227-kg) body of the gorilla, and the 3,000-pound (1,364-kg) body of the elephant are all constructed of 100% raw plant food. I am here to settle your mind and demonstrate to you that great size and strength can be accomplished naturally by humans too.

You have the potential to create the exact body you want. You can restructure and rejuvenate your body by rethink-ing yourself, by grasping on to a wider vision of yourself. De-program your old thought habits and re-program yourself for mind mastery. Send down a different body plan to your sub-conscious mind through affirmations and pictures of your ideal self. With consistency, your body and experience will follow suit.

Anchor and maintain a powerful belief system. The most important pre-requisite for accomplishing any goal and for becoming a vibrant, powerful person is a powerful, undiminished belief that what you are doing is indeed the best way to live. This belief must be the product of your own conclusions. It must be strong enough to carry you through the cyclical lows in the process of attaining your goal. Chance, destiny, and fate cannot circumvent, hinder, or control the firm resolve of the determined. We know nothing until intuition agrees. Half-measures never have and never will achieve the desired results.

As you engage in vigorous exercise, leverage your mind by focusing or meditating on your strength and physique goals. Do not allow yourself to be distracted. Listen to high-energy music that you like while training. I listen to progressive heavy metal music when I train. Some people think heavy metal music is negative and depressing, but it's not. Progressive heavy metal music is powerful! Some high-energy bands I highly recommend listening to while training are: Dream Theater, Queensryche, Symphony X, Nevermore, Yngwie Malmsteen, Fates Warning, and Iron Maiden.

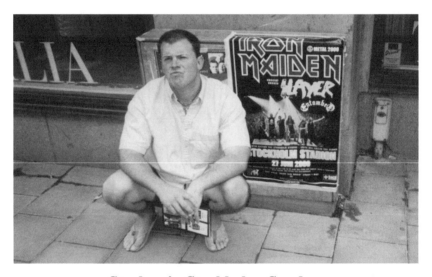

Stephen in Stockholm, Sweden.
The Swedes have great taste in music!

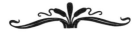

The Raw-Food Diet

*A raw-foodist is not something you become,
it is something that you already are.*
— **Nature's First Law: The Raw-Food Diet**

One of the most important elements of health is diet. Of course food isn't everything, but it is really the foundation upon which everything else is built. Everything that you physically are right now was once the food that went into your mouth, the air you breathed, the water you drank, etc. Other important factors in health are: positive thoughts and associations, sunshine on the skin, empowering relationships, exercise in Nature, interaction with children, interaction with animals (this does not include eating them!), clean air, unpolluted water, and avoidance of mass media.

What we eat deeply and radically affects how we think, feel, and behave. In fact, it directly affects how we interact with our planet. Switching to a raw-food diet has a *massive* positive impact on the environment as well as ourselves. The principle I am describing here is very simple. Life change comes from the inside out. Once you change on the inside, everything changes on the outside.

The most valuable aspect of raw-foodism is its transformative value. You're not the same person just a little bit healthier on The Raw-Food Diet. You become a *radically* new person with new interests, goals, and aspirations. As my long-time friend and business partner David Wolfe says, "We are not really human beings, we are human becomings, because we are constantly becoming something more." How profoundly true!

A major problem that most people have is eating for emotional reasons. Never eat until you are hungry. Every cell and part of your body must be exercised before you eat so that the food you eat will be properly metabolized. Create a demand for the food every time you eat. Earn your food. Even if you put the best food in your body when you are not hungry, the food will not be assimilated at the most efficient level and it will drain energy unnecessarily.

Here are some good guidelines to keep in mind:

1. Do not eat when fatigued.
2. Do not eat immediately before beginning exercise.
3. Do not eat when under mental or physical distress.
4. Do not eat when ill.
5. Do not eat cooked foods.
6. Do not overeat.
7. Do not eat foods containing pesticides.
8. Do not eat unnatural additives, chemicals and/or other synthetic products.

Throw out any and all bread. You cannot build strength on bread. Eating bread makes you as flimsy and as pliable as the bread itself. Bread also contains an enormous amount of estrogen (a female hormone). If you are male, it has the propensity to throw your sexuality way out of whack. I've seen it happen many times, from male breast development to sexual dysfunctions. Stack the odds in your favor by not eating it.

Immediately throw out all medication (pills, liquids, etc.) of any kind. Medications are poisons and the body must go through a tremendous internal crisis to eliminate and detoxify them. A "poison" is anything ingested that cannot be metabolized and utilized effectively by the body, and that the body must waste resources (greater than any benefit received therefrom) on eliminating and/or detoxifying.

Remember, you have to detoxify *all* the toxic waste and poisons out of your body, and keep them out, before you can build up on raw foods. You have to be willing to detoxify *all* the way. Again, you can't clean up the river as long as the chemical plant is dumping waste upstream! Our bloodstreams are our most important rivers. It is possible to gain muscle and unleash strength you never knew you had if you simply adhere to the Laws of Nature.

What people must understand and accept is the fact that for every disciplined effort in life, there are multiple rewards. I've seen people go through very mild detoxifications, and I've seen some pretty hard-core detoxifications. It really depends on how you lived your life before. Someone who was a heavy drug user, medicine taker, or smoker is obviously going to have a heavier detoxification than someone who lived their life more in accordance with the Laws of Nature. The Laws of Nature are there for you to use to your benefit. Human progress through knowledge has been solely and exclusively a chiselling away at the distinctions which define the Laws of Nature. The greatest insights in history have been by those who revealed a new distinction about Nature (which was actually there all along). When the body gets buried in unprocessed residues of cooked foods and finally has the energy to release them, it will. *There is no magic pill, only a magic process.* As we untangle ourselves out of the cooked-food residues, we release suppressed toxins and emotions. Hang in there, understand what is happening, read materials on The Raw-Food Diet, stay active, get outdoors, and enjoy the abundance life has to offer!

Don't worry about detoxification symptoms, they are clear signals that your body is healing.

Fasting is the fastest way to heal the body. A good guideline is to fast one day a week. The problem with raw food is that it actually contains too much nutrition! Giving your body a rest one day a week is great. Newcomers to The Raw-Food Diet need not worry about fasting until they have been 100% raw for at least 6 months. It is best to educate yourself first on the subjects of raw-food diet and fasting and take one step at a time, initially just stopping the intake of cooked food and progressing from there.

Steroids are an abomination. Cooked-eating, meat-eating, pill-popping, steroid-injecting body-builders have false, cooked, artificial strength. They have truly accepted a Faustian bargain (a short-term gain at the expense of a long-term tragedy). Sooner or later, they will have to pay the price. And they do, as we see among most of the retired body-builders and athletes whose bodies have fallen apart by the time they reach the age of fifty.

Eat the foods you like; eat foods that agree with you. Since everyone is a bit different, everyone should eat a bit differently, according to their natural instincts, desires, and environments. Eat only foods which you feel satisfy your nutritive needs, digestibility, and assimilation. What is desirable for you may not be desirable for someone else.

Eating cooked carbohydrates, dead proteins, and burned fats, leads to an internal accumulation of numerous mutagenic (carcinogenic) products caused by the cooking process.

No cooked food is benign. Cooked food acts malignantly by exhausting your bodily energies, inhibiting your healing process, and decreasing your alertness, efficiency, and productivity. When you treat food with thermal fire, you destroy the life-force in it. The heat of cooking destroys vitamins, enzymes, nucleic acids, chlorophyll, de-animates minerals, and damages fats, turning them into dangerous trans-fatty acids. These changed fats are incorporated into the cell wall and interfere with the respiration of the cell, causing an increase in cancer and heart disease. The heat disorganizes the protein structure, leading to a deficiency of the amino acids. The fibrous or woody element of food (cellulose) is changed completely from its natural condition by cooking. When this fibrous element is cooked, it loses its broom-like quality to sweep the alimentary canal clean. Fire destroys, it doesn't create anything. When you add flame to something, it becomes less than it was before. If you don't believe me, try adding flame to your house. Will it become more or less than it was before? Well, the same situation exists with your food. If you add heat or flame to it, it will become less than it was before. The ramifications of cooking are massive.

Eating cooked food suppresses the immune system. After eating cooked foods, the blood immediately shows an enormous increase of leukocytes or white blood cells/corpuscles. The white blood cells are supposedly a first line of defense and are, collectively, popularly called "the immune system." This spontaneous multiplication of white corpuscles always takes place in normal blood immediately after the introduction of any virulent infection or poison into the body since the white corpuscles are the fighting organisms of the blood. There is no multiplication of white corpuscles when raw plant food is eaten. The constant daily fight against the toxic effects of cooked food unnecessarily exhausts the body's strength and vitality, thus causing disease and the modern-day shortness of life.

Ingesting cooked food allows inorganic minerals to enter the blood, circulate through the system, settle in the arteries and veins, and deaden the nerves. After cooking, the body loses its flexibility, arteries lose their pliability, nerves lose their power of conveying expressions, the spinal cord becomes hardened, and the tissues throughout the body contract. In many cases, this dead matter is deposited in the various joints of the body, causing enlargement of the joints. In other cases, it accumulates as concretions in one or more of the internal organs, finally accumulating around the heart valves. A lack of flexibility in any area of life, especially in the physical body, causes premature aging and weakness. The importance of stretching the body and returning the tissues to a natural elasticity cannot be overstated.

Raw foods are easily digested, requiring only 24-36 hours for transit time through the digestive tract, as compared to 40-100+ hours for cooked foods. Prolonged digestion creates putrefaction and disease in the colon. It robs the body of energy which could be directed towards gaining strength. Remember, digestion takes by far more energy than any other internal bodily activity.

On The Raw-Food Diet you will experience the elimination of body odor and halitosis (bad breath). Eating raw will also alleviate allergies because cooked foods irritate the delicate, thin mucus lining in the body and sinuses. Eating raw allows space for free-breathing and a better internal environment for vigorous physical training.

Raw plant food provides you with more strength, stamina, and energy because it has the best balance of water, nutrients, and fiber, which precisely meet your body's needs.

On The Raw-Food Diet, the mind (memory and power of concentration) will be clearer. You will be more alert, think sharply and more logically. Raw foods not only allow you to build a real base of healthy strong muscle tissue, they also allow you to focus more clearly, especially when exercising.

Raw foods will not leave you with a tired feeling after a meal. There is a tendency towards lethargy after a cooked meal. When eating raw foods, you require less total sleep and you will experience more restful sleep. This allows more time to achieve goals and enjoy exercise activities with family and friends.

Raw foods are delectable, delightful, and delicious and have more flavor than cooked foods. Cooked food is dead and bland. That is why people need to doctor-up cooked food with ridiculous additives. These "flavor-enhancing" (stimulating) additives irritate your digestive system and overstimulate other organs. Avoid the following harmful additives: refined sugar, table salt, irradiated spices, and other suspicious condiments.

Nature clearly demonstrates, in the eating habits of every form of life, the basic principles of nutrition. Animals, in their feeding, obtain a balanced intake of basic food components so that the ratio of sugars, fats, proteins, carbohydrates, mineral salts, and vitamins to each other remains basically the same.

The plant is the basis of all animal life on Earth; all animals derive their food either directly or indirectly from plants. Eat raw, fresh, organic fruits and vegetables to supply the requisite vitamins and minerals. Eating these will minimize digestive stress and conserve bodily energy. A minimum of digestive power should be expended in order to obtain a maximum of nutritional return. Again, eat only those foods which you can most readily digest and assimilate.

Eating animals and animal products is unnecessary and can be extremely harmful to your health. All heart disease has been directly linked to the unnatural consumption of animal products and a wide variety of other diseases and ailments also find their basis in the consumption of animal products. But, can you gain strength and muscle without eating meat? Just ask vegetarian Bill Pearl, who won four Mr. Universe body-building titles. Arnold Schwarzenegger once said, "Bill Pearl never talked me into becoming a vegetarian, but he did convince me that a vegetarian could become a champion body-builder."

There are also massive mental repercussions from eating animal products. There is a link between violence and eating animal products. Can you fathom that the primary way in which people on this planet interact with animals is by eating them?!

You most certainly can build muscle on a plant-based diet, especially if you engage in rigorous anaerobic exercise. This is how to build muscle mass. It is funny that people believe you can build muscle out of cooked animal muscle, but not on fruits and green-leafed vegetables! Cooked animal muscle is a dead, lifeless, coagulated substance; raw fruits and vegetables are perfectly designed and contain everything your body requires in a simple, usable form.

My partner in health, David Wolfe, has noted in his book **The Sunfood Diet Success System** that all long-term raw-foodists he has met and/or interviewed eat out of the following classes of foods:

1. Green-Leafy Vegetables (wild greens being
   the best)
2. High-Water-Content Sugar Fruits (melons,
   tropical/subtropical fruits, etc.)
3. Fats (avocados, coconuts, nuts, seeds,
   olives, durians, etc.)

These three food classes form the essentials of The
Raw-Food Diet. These foods balance against each other and
keep you centered. Think of the three food classes as corners
of a triangle, the center being the balance point. For example,
when one eats too many fatty foods, the internal propensity (or
instinct) is to eat more greens and juicy sugar fruits to balance.
If one eats too many juicy sugar fruits, the internal propensity
(or instinct) is to eat more greens and fats to balance. If one
eats too many greens, the internal propensity (or instinct) is to
eat more fats and juicy sugar fruits to balance. Keep this in
mind as you develop a consistent raw-diet which can catapult
you to your maximum potential.

Chlorophyll-rich foods are the blood of life. The
chlorophyllous green, leafy vegetables are the richest sources
of alkaline mineral salts, living carbohydrates, and top-quality
proteins. The most complex laboratory in the world resides in
the photosynthetic green-leaf organs of plants. The leaves contain an excess of organic base compounds in a colloidal form.

For maximum strength and body-building, eat a large
green-leafy salad each day. Organic or home-grown romaine
lettuce or dinosaur kale are two of the most superior leafy-veg-
etables nutritionally and they are the most palatable when eaten
alone. Use also the chlorophyll-rich and mineral-saturated
wild greens such as dandelion, malva (mallow), lamb's quarters, thistle, etc. The more natural your food, the better. Also,
celery (the favorite food of the gorilla) is a fine addition to the

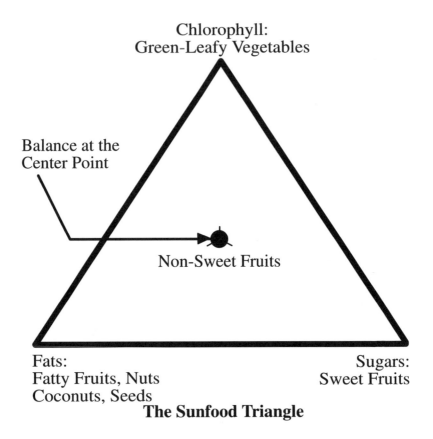

The Sunfood Triangle

body-builder's diet. Celery provides organic sodium which balances out the potassium of fruits, providing a balanced internal chemistry. Cut up an apple or an avocado and mix it with your salad if you find it dry.

Fruits are in many ways our most natural food. Try to eat non-hybridized fruit (fruit with viable seeds) and wild fruit. I do not buy into the "hypoglycemia is caused by fruit" idea, even if it is hybridized commercial fruit. I do believe, from experience, that a good percentage of the fruits you eat should be non-sweet fruits such as cucumber, red bell pepper, tomato, corn, and zucchini. I also believe that fruit causes a cleansing of refined sugars out of the body which may have been stored there for years, even decades. Never eat refined sugar of any kind (that includes the sugar found in bread and other cooked starches). Find one or more staple fruits which you like so much, they make you feel as if you can live off of them alone. I personally prefer melons, berries, and citrus fruits.

Though it is not totally necessary, for ideal digestion, eat one type of fruit at a time. Try not to mix different types of fruits together. Follow a "mono-diet" when eating fruit. Eat foods that are in season (see the Seasonal Produce Availability section on page 203). Eat the heavy fuel or "high-calorie" fruits such as apples, avocados, cherimoyas, dates, durians, grapefruits, lemons, limes (ripe, not green), mangos, etc.

Nuts are also a potent food, especially in the winter season. I do not like to use the word "moderation," but remember to moderate with nuts. You can get "nutted out." Eat nuts with naturally-dried apricots or raisins for superior digestion. My experience has shown that eating dried apricots or raisins and nuts in the winter increases one's resistance to cold weather. Nuts are a heavy food which can provide you with the fuel or calories for long, intense workouts.

Protein is a heavy building material which appears in nuts, but is also available in vegetables and even fruits. Cooked protein is coagulated and dead. Cooked proteins simply clog the tissue system causing the muscle tissue to puff up. Strength is gained at the expense of vitality and the body is put under a tremendous strain to prevent damage to the ligaments and joints. Adequate, raw proteins help you to gain desirable weight, but are not necessary in large amounts.

The gorilla is the strongest land mammal pound-for-pound. A gorilla has the strength equivalent to bench pressing 4,000 pounds (1800 kg)! Gorillas eat primarily green-leafy materials, which are the real body builders. Of course, the gorilla is a 100% raw plant eater! Do you think if a gorilla ate bread, meat, cheese, candy, etc. every day it would be able to perform feats of strength like this? I think not.

Raw proteins are built from substances called amino acids. Of the 22 necessary amino acids, there are eight which our bodies must get from outside sources. All of these eight are present in raw plant foods (especially in green foods) in their correct proportions. Think of a cow which is 1,000+ pounds (450 kg) of protein flesh. What does a cow eat? Grass. All the amino acids necessary for the cow to build an enormous body are present in grass, and any green plant for that matter.

To gain strength and healthy weight, I also recommend sending "hot" food through the intestinal tract on a regular basis. Pick your favorite "hot" raw foods, whether they be: garlic, onions, ripe hot peppers, ginger, radishes, etc. You can juice these foods with vegetables, mix them with salads, or eat them in a mono-meal. "Hot" foods burn out parasites and stimulate the intestines. I have noted that with some people turning on to raw foods, excessive thinness is often associated with parasite infections. Now I know that Natural Hygienists believe these foods to be irritants... and they are irritants... to parasites in your body! I've been to Natural Hygiene conventions and let me tell you, most of the people there look like something out of "Night of the Living Dead." A great axiom to follow is: "Don't listen to anyone, in any field of information, if they are not receiving the results that you desire." You wouldn't go to a beggar on the street for financial advice would you? Well, don't take the advice of out-of-shape, emaciated, sickly, unhealthy people!

Dead food, negative emotions, and inactivity drain your energy and cause weight loss. This becomes definitely more true the closer you get to a 100% raw diet. My experience has indicated that one cannot reach her/his ideal body weight unless the body is significantly purified by a 100% raw-diet. Those who linger close to 100%, but do not actually achieve it will not be able to perfectly gain the weight they desire. One may even gain up to 10 pounds (4.5 kg) by moving from 98% raw food to 100% raw food!

Remember, cooked food (even a small amount) drains and dehydrates your body of precious, heavy, living water. Living water is derived most abundantly from living plants, especially fruit. Living water is not just filtered water which comes through the roots and into the plant; living water is actually created during photosynthesis. Living water is heavier, more electrified, and has greater solubility properties than ordinary water (the hydrogen atoms are pulled together more tightly in each molecule of living water, thus giving the molecule greater polarity).

Living water weighs more on a molecular level than dead tap or spring water (the 60 trillion cells multiplied by the slightly heavier water-weight of every molecule produces a big difference in overall body weight). So you will gain weight on raw food as long as you are 100% raw. I could not gain weight until I went 100% raw. The water stored in my body would go towards diluting and digesting bread and dead food and I would feel drained. Whenever I would eat cooked food I would become sallow and lose 5 to 10 pounds (2.3 to 4.5 kg)! Commit yourself—go 100% raw. It is *not* extreme! Remember, every natural living organism on this planet is a 100% raw-food eater. They aren't 99% raw, they are 100% raw! That's trillion of organisms. Are they all being extreme? I think not.

Also, as a general rule, the higher the water-content of the food, the higher its energy and vibration. The lighter your diet, the more energy you will have. To achieve your desired weight, stabilize the living-water weight level in your body. One's living-water weight will not stabilize until that last jump to a 100% raw-diet (high in fruit and wild greens) is made.

Listed below are two special strategies I have successfully employed to gain healthy weight over the years. Employ them as part of your daily dietary regime and you will see results.

<u>Strategy 1: Coconuts and green juice</u>

I have used the following formula to energize my blood, build my body, and gain 25+ pounds of healthy muscle weight (9+ kg):

I drink two to four coconuts worth of coconut water almost daily. I buy young coconuts (with a soft, jelly-like interior) which are commonly found in Asian-food markets. I scoop out the jelly-like pulp as a meal for myself or my family, or save it for smoothies or coconut custard. I add freshly-made green juice to the coconut water, which saturates my body with usable muscle-building minerals.

This program targets the blood specifically. When you rebuild your blood, you rebuild your body. Coconut water is the closest substance to human blood plasma found in the plant world. Fifty-five percent of the blood is plasma. Green chlorophyll is the closest substance to human hemoglobin in the plant world. Coconut water combined with green juice is a powerhouse way to revitalize the blood and build the body. Ann Wigmore often recommended coconut water mixed with wheatgrass juice, a combination I enjoy as well.

I eat the pulp inside the coco for its incredible raw plant

fat content. Raw plant fats, as I mentioned before, are essential to a powerfully vibrant raw diet. Fats are much more important in the human diet than protein, and fats are also more important for body-building than protein. Raw plant fats lubricate the digestive tract, they are "soft" on the body (easy to assimilate), and they deliver specific protection to the wall of each cell. Fats also provide extra electrons to the cells and thus they are an anti-oxidant.

Here is one of my secret body-building formulas:

CAPTAIN'S POWERHOUSE

In a blender:
1 young coconut (juice and pulp)
1 large avocado
2 handfuls of wild or organic greens

Strategy 2: Eat only once or twice a day.

Eating only once or twice a day is another strategy you can employ to gain strength and muscular weight. Eat large meals when you eat. Note: This is not necessarily the optimal way for everyone to eat, but keep in mind what your goal is here—to gain strength and healthy muscular weight. After you achieve your desired strength and weight, you can return to a more sustainable eating schedule. Here's an example for you. Though Sumo Wrestlers are big, fat, cooked-food eaters, the way they eat to gain weight is interesting and instructive. Sumo Wrestlers fast all day and then, right before they go to bed, they eat a massive cooked meal. What happens is the body "thinks" that there is a shortage of food all day so it conserves energy and the metabolism slows way down. Then, they eat a massive meal right before they go to sleep and the body is not able to process and assimilate most of the food—so they inevitably gain weight (of course not healthy weight though!). It has been my experience that raw-foodists who eat all day are thinner than those who eat once or twice a day. For raw-eaters who eat all day, their bodies "think" that there is an abundance of food coming in so their metabolism speeds up in order to process all the food coming in.

To further illustrate this concept, I will use the following analogy: Anyone familiar with standard weight-training principles knows that to build mass you need to do low-repetition exercises with a heavy weight. And to tone-up, you need to do high-repetition exercises with a light weight. The same principles can be applied to eating for mass or eating to tone-up. High-repetition exercises with a low weight equates to eating a high frequency of small meals throughout the day. You are not able to gain mass by eating this way. Low-repetition exercises with a high weight equates to eating a low frequency of large meals during the day (only one or two meals a day). This is by far the most important aspect of gaining weight and strength on The Raw-Food Diet.

In 1997, I took a 12-day trip to Hawaii. There were so many exotic fruits there, I found myself eating pretty much all day (high frequency of small meals). Guess what? I lost 13 pounds in those 12 days. When I returned home, I ate only at night, lifted weights and took in sunlight during the day and the weight returned quickly.

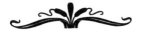

Minerals

I'm goin' bald right now!
— Big Boy

We are made up of minerals. It's really as simple as that. "You are what you eat" is true! A diet high in raw, organic, alkaline minerals is absolutely essential for superior health. A diet lacking in these minerals is distastrous, especially for a bodybuilder. If a little is good, then a lot must be better, right? RIGHT! A good way to make sure you are saturating your body daily with the highest quality raw, organic minerals is by using 1-2 heaping tablespoons of Nature's First Food raw superfood (see page 61). I now supplement my diet with it most every day. The stuff works wonders! It is 100% raw, organic, and vegan. The high silicon content, the probiotics, enzymes, and trace minerals of this superfood make it a great muscle and bone builder.

Sodium

The importance of sodium for bodybuilders cannot be overstated. I recently watched a program in which they did a profile on a popular bodybuilder who said he eats pickles for sodium. Raw olives contain a good sodium content (specifically Raw Power! Olives—they contain celtic sea salt which is particularly high in magnesium and contains over 80 essential trace minerals), are the fruit highest in minerals, and are a much better choice than pickles! Other natural foods high in good, usable sodium are: celery, kale, dandelion, spinach, and sea vegetables (such as laver and dulse).

Traveling

When traveling (or living) in third-world countries or other places where vegetable cleanliness is questionable, I highly recommend taking your Nature's First Food with you. You will be glad you did! Nature's First Food is of course an excellent source of green-vegetable minerals.

Baldness and Hair Re-Growth

Male-pattern baldness has been attributed to a diet low in minerals. Genetic disposition and heredity of course also play a role. In my own personal experience, I started going bald in my mid-20's. I have since grown back some of my hair due to a diet high in raw, organic, alkaline minerals. I also rub **Life Crystal Cream** into my scalp and hair every morning. The healing power of this elixir is incredible! People spend thousands upon thousands of dollars on hair transplants and hair-growth products and the results are usually sad. Life Crystal Cream contains aloe vera, which is rich in monoatomic elements (not many plants are). Also, **Pureganic Liquid Manna** is a product containing platinum-based monoatomic elements suspended in frequency-charged water. These monoatomic elements are the most important of all trace minerals. This product can be taken orally.

If you have not yet read **The Sunfood Diet Success System** by David Wolfe, do yourself a favor and read it! This book describes in detail how to balance minerals, foods, and food classes to achieve specific physical, mental, emotional, and spiritual states. The importance of eating green-leafy vegetables is also made crystal clear.

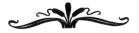

Absorption, Assimilation, and Digestion

It's not only what you eat,
it's what you absorb that counts.
— Dr. Bernard Jensen

If you are having trouble making weight and strength gains, you may have absorption, assimilation, and/or digestion problems. Have you ever known someone (maybe even yourself) who is very thin but eats massive amounts of food? The reason for this phenomenon may be that this person is absorbing very little nutrients due to a layer of "plaque" on her or his intestinal tract. The intestinal villi cannot freely pull in nutrients. This layer inhibits crucial in and outflows of gastric and intestinal fluids. When these flows are hindered, the natural balance is offset, causing a chain reaction of nasty problems such as: a vitamin B-12 deficiency, diverticulitis, candida, leaky bowel syndrome, colitis, cysts and tumors.

The process of perfect absorption, assimilation, digestion, and elimination is the great secret of life. The better your absorption, assimilation, and digestion, the less you need to eat. Another essential word of advice is to chew foods very well and eat slowly. Fletcherize your food. Dr. Fletcher taught that each mouthful of food should be chewed at least 50 times before swallowing. An ancient Indian proverb states: "Chew your food well, for the stomach has no teeth." Thoroughly mix the food with your saliva. The more your food is ground up and chewed, the greater will be the absorption by the body.

Lack of intestinal absorption is a major reason why people have trouble gaining weight.

Typically, the cooked-food eater's intestinal tract is lined with a mucus layer which prevents nutriments from passing through the intestinal villi. This mucus must be broken up and dissolved to restore the proper functioning of the intestinal tract. I recommend a series of colon irrigations to jump-start the cleansing process. Also, there are certain foods which efficiently dissolve mucus, such as the fig. The fig is ranked as one of the highest mucus dissolvers in Ragnar Berg's Table in Arnold Ehret's book **Mucusless Diet Healing System**.

Of course, raw-plant foods improve the total inner environment. Raw food greatly enhances the efficiency of nutrient absorption. Over time, The Raw-Food Diet enables the body to dislodge and remove accumulated wastes from the intestinal folds.

For mild cases of poor absorption, assimilation, and/or digestion, I recommend occasionally eating the cassia fruit. Cassia is the pod-fruit of a tree that is found in tropical regions. Cassia is a natural laxative which can play a crucial role in the early stages of a raw food diet in order to facilitate the detoxification processes and to help alleviate constipation. Cassia discs are contained within the pod of the fruit. Each disc tastes like a cross between chocolate and carob and can be sucked on until it dissolves. Five to six discs should be enough to help with bowel movements. Each pod contains 40+ discs.

For severe cases of poor absorption, assimilation, and/or digestion, I highly recommend the EJUVA Herbal-Intestinal Cleanse. Having debated these issues for many years and worked with thousands of people, I highly recommend this herbal-intestinal cleanse program for anyone who experiences absorption, assimilation, and/or digestion problems. This is a 4-6 week herbal program involving increasing the intake of herbs and juices and decreasing the intake of food. Certain herbs contain compounds (especially when eaten in conjunction with each other) which force the digestive system to release mucoid plaque (encrusted mucus created by a lifetime of eating cooked foods, animal foods, medicine, etc.). These herbs are more effective in removing intestinal plaque than any green-leafy vegetable, fruit, or juice combination we have found. It is common to see mucoid plaque come out of people who have been eating 100% raw foods for over 3 years. Mucoid plaque is very difficult to relieve unless one is doing raw foods, juices and herbs. The Ejuva cleanse is 100% raw, 100% organic or wild, contains no fillers, no isolated compounds, no bentonite (bentonite has been shown to contain 22% aluminum), is 100% naturally dried, cut, sifted, and compressed into three different tablet formulations to be chewed up like food. Also included in the cleanse program are: a psyllium/flax/chia seed mix for juices while on the cleanse and a probiotic formulation. Simple, detailed instructions on how to follow the cleanse are included. This herbal intestinal rebuilding kit is a little pricey, but worth every penny. Call 1-800-205-2350 and mention Raw Power! to get a $20 discount!

Vitamin B-12 Deficiency

A vitamin B-12 deficiency can arise when there is a complete disruption in the human body's intestinal flora. In a normal situation vitamin B-12 is absorbed from bacteria in the intestinal tract. Most meat eaters are not afflicted by this deficiency because animal flesh (including insect tissue) contains a plethora of B-12. Maintaining adequate B12 levels on a raw-food diet can be done by consuming Vita Synergy multi-vitamin, Nature's First Food, sea vegetables, blue-green algae, spirulina and especially freshly-picked unwashed food (which provides the intestines with soil-based organisms which are transmutated in good intestinal flora which help create excellent B12 levels). Also, excessive amounts of sweet fruit in the diet can cause the intestinal flora to become sterilized (sugar is an antibiotic). Eat more greens and drink more green juices. Get out in the sun as much as possible. Chlorinated tap water also sterilizes food.

Two raw-food books that discuss the subject of B12 are **The Sunfood Diet Success System** by David Wolfe and **Conscious Eating** by Dr. Gabriel Cousens.

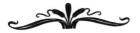

Exercise and Weight Training

Come on, let's get serious.
— Arnold Schwarzeneggar

Total fitness has three vital components: Aerobic Conditioning, Flexibility, and Muscular Conditioning.

Aerobic activity is anything that uses up a lot of oxygen. Oxygen is delivered to the muscles by the cardiovascular system—the lungs, heart, and circulation of the blood. The system is developed by continuous, high-repetition exercise such as running, swimming, jumping rope, riding a bicycle, etc.

Muscles, tendons, and ligaments tend to shorten over a period of time, which limits our range of motion and renders us more vulnerable to injury when sudden stresses are placed on these body parts. But we can counteract this tendency by stretching exercises and physical stretching programs.

The best way to develop and strengthen the muscles is resistance training. When you contract the muscles against resistance, they adapt to this level of effort. The best and most efficient way of doing this is through weight training.

To gain strength and muscular weight, do progressive, anaerobic exercise six days a week, giving yourself one day off. Push yourself—be physical! And think *powerfully*. Remember, the Mind is the most important factor.

Both men and women can build beautiful sculpted muscles through intense resistance exercise. Remember, 50% of the body's weight is muscle.

Muscles, as their growth is promoted, provide the ground-work for genuine physical beauty. The more your muscles grow, the more beautiful you become. Bodily form and the perfect figure can be developed by muscular development, sunshine on the skin, deep-breathing, and proper control of weight by eating naturally and sensibly.

To improve your balance to an unimaginable level, lift weights standing up on one foot at a time. Experiment! You'll find that your form and lifting mechanics sharpen up dramatically.

Do the vigorous exercises you feel good doing. Do exercises which agree with you. You can exercise anywhere. Exercise whenever you watch television, listen to the radio, or audio tapes, etc., but be on guard against the negative, hypnotic suggestion of mass media. Keep in mind that participating in mass media contributes to a negative attitude and a negative outlook on life, so avoid it whenever possible. When we were teenagers, David Wolfe, my brother Scott and I used to pass a dumbbell back and forth while we watched a video, doing sets of exercises until the video was over.

To gain maximum weight and to build muscular size or strength, you must perform exercise feats which you are not presently capable of doing. You must attempt the momentarily impossible. Such attempts should involve maximum efforts against resistance. This is what separates success from failure.

Do exercises which are progressively stressful or resistant. Do exercises which are difficult yet safe, which you enjoy, and which suit your life-style. Preferably, exercise outdoors under the sun or, in the alternative, at a convenient facility. Exercise at a convenient time of day or night, as long and as frequently as possible, and as regularly as possible. Choose a program you will follow throughout your life. Exercise every part of your body as vigorously as possible. Be aware of each body part. Exercise until the resulting fatigue relaxes you.

Start your exercise program with amounts of weight and repetitions which are easy to perform. Advance gradually and increase slowly. Muscles should be contracted to their fullest extent and joints should be carried through their full range of movement. Place demands on your body within reasonable limits. Once the muscles are warmed up, then conduct short periods of intense, vigorous, extremely resistant exercise. This will put more muscle weight on your body than maintaining a long period of mild exercise.

To gain weight, do more anaerobic (without oxygen) exercises than aerobic (with oxygen) exercises in your workout. Aerobic exercise is good for your heart and helps you gain endurance, not muscular development.

A fantastic exercise is swimming underwater, or doing underwater laps in a pool. Swimming is an aerobic activity, but when you swim underwater while holding your breath, you greatly increase your lung capacity, which will help your weightlifting work-out. You will see a big difference in your breathing after a few weeks of doing the exercise consistently.

Aerobic exercises are light exercises such as: walking, jogging, long-distance running, dancing, long-distance swimming, long-distance cycling, cross-country skiing, etc.

To gain weight and develop muscles, do anaerobic exercises. Anaerobic exercises are heavy exercises such as: lifting

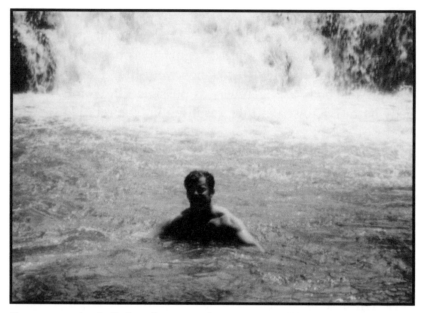

I recommend doing laps under water whilst holding your breath. Also, treading water for 30 minutes after an intense work-out really gives your body an extra boost and gives you an edge over everyone else!

heavy weights, low-repetition concentrated weight-lifting, arm-wrestling, sprinting, wrestling, rope climbing, jumping, speed cycling, sprint swimming, etc.

Anaerobic exercises are intense exercises which can only be tolerated for a few moments. They are short bursts of high-energy activities. They use muscle groups at high intensities which exceed the body's capacity to use oxygen to supply energy. They create an oxygen debt by using energy produced without oxygen. They are activities which demand such a great muscle explosion that the body has to rely upon an internal metabolic process for oxygen.

Breathe between anaerobic exertions. Take deep,

diaphragmatic breaths. Anaerobic exercises may be: isotonic, isokinetic, isometric, and/or negative or "eccentric" exercises.

Isotonic exercise involves movement of a constant heavy weight through a full range of possible movement. It is a muscular action in which there is a change in the length of the muscle, while the tension remains constant. The bench press is a classic example of an isotonic exercise.

Isokinetic exercise is exercise in which there is accommodation resistance and constant speed. Nautilus is a type of isokinetic machine where the machine varies the amount of resistance being lifted to match the force curve developed by the muscle. Isokinetics is exercising in which the maximum force of which the muscle is capable of is applied throughout the range of motion.

Isometric exercise involves a static contraction. It is the application of a high percentage of your existing strength against an unmoving resistance, a fixed limit. Isometrics entails pushing against an immovable force such as: another set of opposing muscles, a wall, building, door, bar, taught rope, towel, two-ton truck, etc. If you push hard enough, you feel stress on your muscles. In isometrics, each exercise should be practiced at several joint angles. Training at many angles distributes the strength gains throughout the range of the muscle's movement. In isometrics, each "all-out" push or pull should be held as long as possible, to the point of muscular failure. Isometric exercises can be done practically anywhere. They are simple and effective. Isometrics increase the strength and improve the muscles' tone and shape. Isometric exercise entails muscular contraction where the muscle maintains a constant length and the joints do not move.

In negative or "eccentric" exercises, you lower the

weight very slowly, at a smooth, steady pace, without interrupting the downward movement. In positive or "concentric" exercise, you raise the weight at normal speed. In negative exercise, your muscle is stretching and lengthening while maintaining tension against resistance. In positive exercise, the muscle is contracting and shortening against resistance. In negative exercise, you resist pressure and in positive exercise, you apply pressure. The muscle has the ability to handle more force during negative exercise than it can during positive exercise. For example, when performing a bench press, the positive part of the repetition is the portion during which the weight is being pressed from the chest to arm's length. The negative portion of the repetition is the part during which the weight is lowered back down to the chest. In negative pull-ups, you climb into the top position using your legs, so that you simply lower yourself back down. Negative parallel bar dips can be done in the same way.

All four of these anaerobic exercise types: isotonic, isokinetic, isometric, and/or negative or "eccentric" should be employed as part of your workout program.

My personal exercise program is one that combines weight-training and yogic principles. These principles include: focused, intentional breathing, prolonged muscular contractions (known as asanas or "poses" in yoga practice), correct posture and alignment, and deep relaxation. All have been incorporated into my weight-training program to form the most intense fitness program anywhere in the world today.

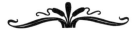

Sunshine

*Separation from sunlight will result in disease, just as
surely as will separation from fresh air, food, and water.*
— Dr. Zane Kime

The human organism is solar-powered. All life on this
spinning planet is sustained directly or indirectly by the sun.

If you want to build muscle and strength, it is important
to get out into the sun. The sun is the source of all life on Earth.
Sunlight quickens the detoxification process and lays a solid
foundation for healing and muscle-building by pulling toxins, in
a magnetic fashion, out of the muscle tissue to the surface of
the skin for elimination.

A common myth is that the sun causes skin cancer. The
sun doesn't cause skin cancer, the sun causes all life on Earth!
Skin cancer is caused by toxicity within the body. When this
toxicity is detoxified through the skin (our largest eliminative
organ), it is sometimes "baked" onto the skin, bringing forth a
cancer condition. Blaming the sun for skin cancer is like blaming fresh air for lung cancer.

You must have internal protection from the sun's rays in
the form of proper, natural, raw-food nutrition. External "protection" like sunscreen is an abomination. The same internal
mechanism that keeps a plant from burning up under the hot sun
can keep you from sunburning. A plant is in direct sunlight for
hours upon hours every day of its existence. A plant dries up
and dies when it no longer has the internal protection that it

requires. The second best protection from sunburn is knowing when to retreat to shade for a rest.

Bask in the sun and get outside for exercise every day! You cannot gain strength and healthy weight if you are sitting indoors all day. The best place to exercise is not in an artificial, air-conditioned gym, but in the green outdoors among the living plants, wild animals, and fresh air. If you want to lift heavy weights, bring them outside and exercise in the open air with the sky above. If you feel you can do without them, do not wear shoes, gloves, or belts. Lift weights without clothing if possible. "Gymnasium" means "to train in the nude." However, always keep in mind your own safety when engaged in these activities.

Sunbathe and airbathe (get fresh, clean air over all the pores of your skin) in the nude. Sunlight and fresh air aid the nutritive processes of the body. You will never feel better than when your body is in shape and you have a good color to your skin. Thinness is associated with paleness. I have also found that people who are afraid of fruit are usually afraid of the sun and afraid of exercise. So, eat fruit, get out in the Sun, and exercise!

It you live where skies are often overcast, or winters are cold and long, it is still important to get outside every day. Some sunlight can almost always get through cloud cover and a little bit of sunshine on your face every day will make a big difference.

When the body is warmed up by the sun, the tissues expand. Thus, you may find in the summer it is easier to gain strength and weight under the hot summer sun.

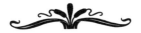

Meditation / Relaxation

Protest the war that's being waged inside your mind.
— David Wolfe

Have you ever known someone who could not, to put it bluntly, just shut up for 60 seconds? Someone who just could not sit still? Someone who needed constant outside stimulation? I once knew a girl who could not close her eyes for 60 seconds. She could not sit still for 30 seconds. And she could not keep her mouth shut for 10 seconds! She was truly the proverbial "runaway headless chicken." As amusing as this sounds, it is extremely detrimental to one's health to not be able to sit calmly with one's eyes closed and mouth shut, thus emptying one's mind of "chatter."

Meditation is not an obscure Indian method, it is not simply a technique, it is a way of being. Meditation is the greatest adventure the human mind can undertake. It is when you are not doing anything at all. Meditation is not something you can do or practice. It is really just a state in which your mind is completely void of any thought, your body completely void of any movement, and your persona void of any emotion.

This emptying of the mind is wonderful and liberating. It is invigorating and it prepares you to re-enter the world fresh and focused. I have found it to be an essential part of my body-building program. One's mind must be clear and fucused to perform potentially dangerous feats of strength.

The best book I've come across on this subject is entitled **Meditation: The First And Last Freedom** by Osho. It is a practical guide for one who desires to quiet the chatter of the mind and achieve self-mastery. This stunningly powerful book is always in the top five most-recommended books by me in my business.

A really cool thing to try if you are adventurous is a meditation session in a floatation tank. In my opinion, floating is the doorway to profound relaxation and altered states. Your mind and body can experience a sensory overload from daily life and a floatation tank can help you maintain your equilibrium by freeing your mind and body. Basically, what happens is the odorless tank is void of light and sound, so your smell, sight, and hearing senses are relieved. The tank's water is filled with hundreds of pounds of Epsom salt to make you 100% bouyant. This will relieve you of your sense of gravity and, in turn, will begin the process of reversing the harmful effects of gravity. The water is heated to your exact body temperature, relieving you of all sense of temperature. You are in the tank for an hour or so. You enter into a different realm of being. I've done it a few times and it is truly an amazing experience. I came out of there a new person, no doubt about it.

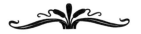

Raw Bodybuilding Foods

Following is a list, unlike any you've seen before, of raw bodybuilding foods. The unknowing person would look at this list and say, "That's rabbit (or chipmunk or bird) food!" but we know better. The first part of the list includes foods that we distribute at Nature's First Law (NFL). The food items in the second part of the list can be acquired at your local food co-op or health-food store, unless otherwise specified.

Part I – Raw Foods Available from Nature's First Law

OLIVES

What if there was something that was 100% natural that would increase your strength and give you instant and blazing energy to get through your workouts? The best raw bodybuilding food on Earth is the olive. Olives are in fact "my Dianabol." Who needs steroids when olives are available? Olives are also the number one mucus-dissolving fruit and the fruit highest in minerals. There are four types of olives that I have found to work best. They are:

Sun-Ripened Greek Olives — These are raw, free-grown, sun-ripened with cold-pressed extra-virgin olive oil and light sea salt. They are fabulous moist olives!

Kalamata-Style Olives (aka Raw Power! Olives) — These raw, free-grown delicious reddish/brown olives are packed in pure water with a dash of fresh garlic, a dash of fresh oregano, one ripe cayenne pepper, and a dash of celtic sea salt.

Italian Black Olives — These raw, free-grown delicious ripe black olives are packed in pure water, a dash of fresh garlic, a dash of fresh oregano, one ripe cayenne pepper, and a dash of celtic sea salt.

Moroccan Olives — Also raw, free-grown, and delicious. These ripe black olives have a rich, full taste.

STONE-PRESSED OLIVE OIL

Olive oil is also quite powerful and is an essential in the raw, living-foods kitchen. The best olive oil is raw, free-grown, **stone-pressed olive oil.** This olive oil is made from ripe olives that are crushed and ground with stone presses using the original techniques developed by the Greeks and Romans thousands of years ago. This oil is true to the original varieties available in the Mediterranean.

RAW ORGANIC NUTS

Nuts are high in minerals and fat, both crucial to muscle building and overall health. Nuts also give you a grounded and full feeling. NFL offers **macadamia nuts, almonds, hazelnuts, pistachios, walnuts, and pecans**, all in-shell to ensure freshness. NFL is North America's only source of **truly raw shelled cashews**. Cashews are the nut of choice for most raw-food chefs.

NUT AND SEED BUTTERS

Raw, organic, **almond butter** is a treat few can resist. It is a very heavy, powerful food. It is also considered a "convenience food" by raw-foodists. I know a guy who is in sales and he travels all over. He always has a jar of almond butter and a spoon in his car. If he ever gets stuck in traffic or is far from home or another food source, he just digs into his almond butter! My wife Jolie usually makes nut milk from "scratch," but when she's pressed for time, she makes nut milk from almond butter. She uses one half of a jar of almond butter (about 3/4 C), 1-5 large pitted dates, and 3 cups of water. She blends them all in the Vita-Mix and has almost instant nut milk! **Pumpkin Seed Butter** is one of the most delicious and nutritious treats you will ever taste. It tastes like peanut butter but is much healthier.

COCONUT OIL/BUTTER

Raw coconut oil/butter is an instant energy source, contains no cholesterol (and has actually been found to lower cholesterol), no trans-fatty acids, and is not hydrogenated. Contrary to commercial oil industry propoganda, unprocessed coconut oil is a very good dietary fat source. Coconut oil is actually lower in calories than most other oils and a little goes a long way.

SEEDS

Like nuts, seeds are mineral rich and high in fat and are filling and satisfying. **Pumpkin seeds** are one of the most important seeds for muscle building. In addition to having many other health benefits, they contain myosin, the main protein that makes up almost all the muscles in the body and plays an important role in muscular contraction. **Hemp seeds** are high in complete protein, bountiful in essential fatty acids, and they taste great (something like a cross between sesame seeds and peanuts.) NFL offers shelled pumpkin and hemp seeds.

Most everyone interested in health and nutrition is now familiar with the health benefits of flax seeds. Rich in essential fatty acids, dietary fiber and lignans, flax seeds have been found to protect heart and artery functions, build the immune system, soothe intestinal problems, relieve constipation, aid in detoxification, balance estrogen levels (comparable to soy), reduce arthritic and other inflammation... the list goes on and on. See the recipe section for ideas on how to add flax to your diet (especially the flax cracker recipes). Nature's First Law also carries a wide variety of **raw, organic flax crackers**.

SUN-DRIED FRUIT

Sun-dried fruit is high in minerals and energizing fruit sugars. My favorite sun-dried fruit, apricots, are especially high in magnesium and potassium, minerals that supply us with energy, stamina, and endurance. They contain iron for blood building and silicon for healthy skin and hair. Nature's First Law offers sun-dried **apricots, calimyrna and black mission figs, jackfruits, mangoes, and raisins (with small seeds)**.

BERRIES

Berries are high in vitamins and minerals and they taste great. Bears eat massive amounts of berries as part of their diet and they gain massive weight and strength from doing so. One type of berries called **goji berries** are perhaps the most nutritionally dense fruit on the planet. They contain 18 kinds of amino acids (six times higher than bee pollen) and contain all eight essential amino acids. Goji berries contain up to 21 trace minerals and are the richest source of carotenoids of all known foods on earth! They contain 500 times the amount of vitamin C, by weight, than oranges, making them second only to camu camu berries as the richest vitamin C source. They are also high in vitamins B1, B2, B6, and E. Goji berries contain polysaccharides which fortify the immune system. One polysaccharide found in this fruit has been found to be a powerful secretagogue (a substance that stimulates the secretion of rejuvenative human growth hormone by the pituitary gland). Goji berries have been traditionally regarded as a longevity, strength-building, and sexual potency food of the highest order.

SEAWEEDS

The health benefits of seaweeds (also becoming known as sea vegetables) are numerous. They are loaded with minerals and trace elements and are a great source of healthful sodium. Nature's First Law offers:

Dulse — Dulse is a red seaweed with flat, fan-shaped fronds that grows from the temperate to frigid zones of the Atlantic and Pacific. Dulse makes a great addition to salads. This alkaline vegetable is an excellent source of iron and many trace minerals. It also contains iodine and manganese, which activate enzyme systems.

Laver (Nori) — Nori (also called Laver) is a dark red, lavender seaweed. It can be added to salads or is great to snack on as-is. Nori has the highest protein contents of any seaweed (48% of dry weight). It also contains an enzyme that helps break down cholesterol deposits. Nori is high in Vitamins A, B1, B3 (niacin), and trace minerals.

Nori Sheets — This raw, sun-dried nori has been processed into thin sheets which can be used to make nori rolls and other raw-food treats (see recipes on pages 126-127).

BEE POLLEN

Bee pollen is the pollen produced by flowers that honey bees gather and bring back to the hive. Pollen grains are microscopic in size and bees collect millions of these individual grains and connect them with nectar into small pellets.

Nature's First Law's beekeepers in New Zealand use a collection device that harvests the bee pollen pellets as the bees return to the hive. The bees are never harmed, and sufficient pollen gets through to provide for the hive's needs. These bees are treated with integrity, ethics, and love. Bee pollen is an alkaline food considered by many nutritionists to be the most complete food found in nature. It is a rich source of high-quality protein and contains all essential amino acids and an abundance of minerals, making it a great strength-builder and brain food. Some of the benefits of bee pollen consumption include: increased energy and stamina, increased muscle growth and definition, immune system fortification, antioxidant activity, enhanced sexuality, and smoothed wrinkles. **Nature's First Law Bee Pollen** is by far the higest-quality and most rigorously-tested bee pollen on the market today.

RAW FOOD ENERGY BARS

Raw Food Energy Bars are the raw-foodist's solution to Power Bars. They're so much better tasting and much better for you! They are raw, minimally-processed, great-tasting and made without additives. They're 100% raw food and high in fiber. Ingredients: bananas, dates, raisins, walnuts, lemon juice. Invest in a case of these bars and watch your energy skyrocket during your workouts.

Part II – Raw Foods Available from your Local Food Co-op or Natural Food Store

GREENS, GREENS, GREENS

I can't say enough about what building foods green leafy vegetables are, so I'll just let them speak for themselves. Dandelion greens, kale, chard, watercress, spinach, collard greens, arugula, endive, parsley, romaine lettuce, mustard greens...

CELERY

I heard someone recently say that celery is devoid of any nutrition and is a "lower vegetable," whatever that's supposed to mean. On the contrary, celery is one of the most nutritious foods on the planet and is an important building food. Jay Kordich, The Juiceman, calls celery the "powerhouse of life-giving nutrition." Celery is high in water, so it replaces valuable fluids lost in sweat. Celery/apple juice has the perfect sodium-potassium ratio (1:5) which is all-important to prevent and relieve muscle cramping and fatigue (see page 149).

CABBAGE

Cabbage is often overlooked as it is not dark green and many people have memories of the putrid smell of cooked cabbage. Cabbage has sometimes been called the king of the cruciferous family. It is highly alkalinizing, cleansing, and rejuvenating and contains substantial amounts of sulfur, iodine, iron, Vitamins C and E and is loaded with the amino acid glutamine. It also happens to be one of the least expensive vegetables. (See recipes for cabbage on pages 120-121, 152.)

COCONUTS

If **young coconuts** are not available at your food co-op or natural food store, check the Asian markets near you or visit the Nature's First Law store in San Diego, California. These are the young, fresh coconuts and are white on the outside. The brown hairy things you see are usually old and dry.

GRAINS

Even though they are traditionally thought of as starchy foods, some grains can add a substantial amount of protein to one's diet when they are sprouted. As opposed to the breakdown of cooked grains, the complex carbohydrates in sprouted grains, along with their available protein, break down into simpler sugars and readily absorbed amino acids. Whole grains are also a source of vegetable lignans, those great anti-cancer, hormone balancing, health-promoting phytochemicals. See the beginning of the recipe section for more information.

**Raw Bodybuilding Foods
are available from Nature's First Law
www.rawfood.com
800-205-2350**

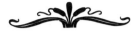

Raw Bodybuilding Supplements

We mock what we do not understand.

I used to be 100% against supplements because of the synthetic nature of them and the fact that the vast majority of them are low-quality abominations. Things have since changed. Due to the negative reputation of supplements perpetuated by the ever-growing raw-food and natural-living communities and the subsequent pressure put on supplement companies to produce high-quality products, there are now some really good raw bodybuilding supplements on the market today. I have found the following supplements to be of high-quality, high integrity, and very helpful to the health and strength seeker:

Nature's First Food is the most nutrient-dense, mineral-rich superfood product ever created. It was developed exclusively for Nature's First Law by one of the world's leading superfood authorities. Nature's First Food has been formulated with a unique understanding of lifeforce energy, enyzmes, raw foods, Mother Nature, and true science. Designed to be taken on a daily basis as part of one's bodybuilding or cleansing program, it contains 100% raw, organic or wildcrafted superfoods, the best probiotic formulation ever put together (designed to implant good bacteria in the intestines), soil organisms, and a full digestive enzyme complex. It is neutral tasting, easily dissolvable and can be added to smoothies and juices. It contains *no fillers* and comes in a amber glass bottle with a metal lid and oxygen absorber for optimum nutrient preservation.

Nature's First Food is more like a meal than a supplement. The mineral density of the foods used in this product is around 24%. A "very high" rating is 17% and average is 8-12%! The dominant mineral in this mix is silica. This was done on purpose because our research has shown that silica is actually the most important alkaline mineral and the mineral that seems to be most deficient in the general population and even among raw-foodists. Silica is found predominately in horsetail, nettles, nopal cactus, dandelions, etc. Silica has extraordinary properties (more than I could explain here). Just to give you an idea, silica is the mineral that crystals are made of.

The probiotics and soil organisms in this product are made of a blend that we trademarked. They are *by far* the best probiotics ever put together in any product of any kind. The probiotic mix in this product is so far ahead of its time, there is no other product that even compares (it is like a Rolls Royce versus a Volkswagon Bug). Probiotics eliminate gas, increase digestive strength, increase counts of all B vitamins, including B12, eat away mucoid plaque, increase vital energy, radically attack and overwhelm fungus, yeast, mold, and candida in the body, help increase assimilation of nutrients, and much more.

Following are Nature's First Food Ingredients (100% raw and organic/wildcrafted superfoods). Land vegetables: whole leaf barley grass, whole leaf wheat grass, nettle leaf, shavegrass (horsetail), alfalfa leaf juice, dandelion leaf juice, kamut grass juice, barley grass juice, oat grass juice, broccoli juice, kale juice, spinach juice, parsley juice, burdock root, nopal cactus, ginger, amla berry. Algaes: spirulina, broken cell wall chlorella. Wildcrafted aquatic vegetables: Icelandic kelp, Nova Scotia dulse. Enzyme Complex: amylase, lipase, protease, cellulase, bromelain, papain. Full complement of probiotics. 100% superfoods, no fillers. As you can see, this is the world's best superfood diet supplement or meal replacement.

Pure Synergy is another fantastic superfood blend of 60 different plants, herbs, and superfoods. This product was developed and perfected over a 20-year period by Mitchell May, PhD. It was originally conceived to help Mitchell May recover from a severe car accident that caused extreme nerve and tissue damage. Pure Synergy is one of the only superfood products that can rival Nature's First Food in quality and effect.

Healthforce Spirulina is 65% protein, the highest source of protein found in any plant food (it contains all 8 essential amino acids). Spirulina is the world's highest known plant-source of vitamin B-12 and also includes vitamins A, B-1, B-2, B-6, E, K, chlorophyll, cell salts, phytonutrients, and enzymes. The ancient Aztecs thrived on spirulina from Lake Texcoco in Mexico. I have found Healthforce Spirulina to be of the highest quality and highest integrity of all the spirulina products I have tested. It is contained in an oxygen resistant amber glass jar. No pesticides are used in its growth. This spirulina is the best product of its kind on the market today. Goes great with young coconut juice!

MSM (Methyl-Sulfonyl-Methane) is a naturally-occur-ring form of dietary sulfur found in fresh raw foods that are involved in the cycle of rain. MSM is deficient in foods grown in greenhouses or in foods grown through conventional irriga-tion. MSM is fragile and is destroyed by cooking. In the body, MSM softens leathery internal tissues by rebuilding connective tissue with elastic sulfur bonds. This how MSM lives up to its reputation of building collagen and maintaining healthy joints. This is also why MSM increases flexibility (good for yoga and bodybuilding), hastens recovery time from sore muscles, and is excellent for recovery from athletic injuries. Because of its collagen-building properties, MSM creates smooth skin, thick lustrous hair, and strong nails.

Liver Rescue — Keeping the liver healthy is essential to good health. Most peoples' livers are quite weakened due to poor diets and lifestyle choices. One of the liver's functions is to filter toxic materials from the blood, and if it is not functioning at an optimum level, one's health can be compromised. Liver Rescue contains ingredients shown to support liver function. Much research has shown one specific ingredient, milk thistle, to protect the liver from the damaging effects of a wide variety of common toxins, including alcohol. Milk thistle extract is so powerful it has been reported to counteract even overdoses of otherwise lethal drugs.

Pure Radiance C is the highest-quality 100% wholefood vitamin C in the world, providing 200% of the RDI. Deep within the Amazon Rainforest grows a remarkable plant whose berries are an astonishing source of naturally occurring vitamin C—camu camu. Gram for gram, these berries provide over twice as much vitamin C as acerola berries and 30 to 60 times more vitamin C than oranges!

Vita Synergy is the finest multi-vitamin on the market today. I noticed a very positive difference in my well-being the first day of taking it. Vita Synergy is not only one of the first 100%-natural multi-vitamin and mineral products, it is also the first truly 100%-natural tablet. Within its ingredients, you won't find any additives, lubricants, flow agents, glues, synthetic coatings, or chemicals with names you can't pronounce. Vita Synergy is also great for people concerned with B12 issues—it contains over 3,000% of the recommended daily value of vitamin B12! For full details and a complete nutri-

tional breakdown of this amazing new product, please see the following website:
http://www.rawfood.com/vitasynergy.html

Tocotrienols (Super Vitamin E) — This balanced whole food provides a stable variety of essential nutrients necessary to properly fuel a healthy body. Providing a full protein complement, this raw rice bran whole-food complex is highly beneficial for those who require a boost to their nutritional protocol. Tocotrienols contain vitamins, minerals, and essential fatty acids necessary to enhance health. They are the most potent form of antioxidant vitamin E available and a rich source of B vitamins. Tocotrienols were at one time more than $4,000 a bottle in alternative cancer clinics! Great to include in smoothies.

Beauty Antioxidants are chewable caplets that contain grape seed extract, grape skin extract, green tea extract, coastal white pine extract, bilberry, alpha tocotrienols, gamma tocotrienols, carotenoids, as well as co-enzymes Q6-Q10. This array of antioxidants provides incredible free radical protection. Free radical damage has been implicated in accelerating aging, wrinkles, and skin deterioration. Beauty Antioxidants provide internal protection from sun over-exposure. Because we are exposed to 10 times as much radiation as normal during jet air travel, Beauty Antioxidants are also of great value when flying. Beauty Antioxidants also decrease free radical damage caused by environmental toxins, cooked food, and breathing polluted air. Nearly all antioxidants on the market today are extracted in 15 minutes using harsh chemical solvents. The antioxidants in this product are extracted naturally over a period of two weeks.

E3Live: Earth's Essential Elements — This excellent whole raw frozen liquid blue-green algae is rich in nutrients, protein, amino acids, minerals, and chlorophyll. Blue-green algae has been called "nature's most basic food." It can help to purify the blood, promote intestinal regularity and naturally help heal the body. People who eat E3 report increased and sustained energy levels, alertness, and a strengthened immune system. Supplementing your diet with a teaspoon or more of E3Live each day can ensure optimum nutrition. Veteran algae eaters notice the difference right away, and those trying algae for the first time are experiencing the amazing benefits of this nutrient-dense raw food. All are impressed by the vitality and purity of E3Live. E3Live retains the vitality, purity and energy of the fresh, live algae. A special proprietary method preserves life-force and nutritional properties without freeze drying, heat, alcohol, or juice concentrate glycerin. E3Live is harvested in the center of Upper Klamath Lake, far from towns and other possible pollutants. Algae is harvested below the surface of the lake, where it is less likely to have been damaged by the sun. E3Live is only harvested when conditions are optimal and the algae are hearty and flourishing. It is certified organic. Raw-food physician and noted author Gabriel Cousens, M.D. said about E3Live, "There is no other blue-green algae that is as alive and active as E3Live. Of all the algae preparations coming out of Klamath Lake, E3Live has the strongest positive effects."

**All Raw Bodybuilding Supplements
are available from Nature's First Law
www.rawfood.com
800-205-2350**

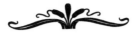

Questions and Answers
with Stephen Arlin

Over the years I've been asked *a lot* of questions pertaining to The Raw-Food Diet and Lifestyle. In this section, I've listed some of the most frequently-asked questions and my answers.

Part I: The Raw-Food Diet

*　　　*　　　*　　　*　　　*

Q: What exactly is The Raw-Food Diet, how do you define raw-foodism, and what does someone have to do, in practice, to be a raw-foodist?

A: Some people consider The Raw-Food Diet the next step past a vegetarian or vegan diet, but it really transcends all diets. It is simply the natural way to nourish your body. A raw-foodist is not something one becomes; a raw-foodist is something that all living creatures on earth already are. We are designed to eat raw foods. Food in its raw, natural state cannot be nutritionally improved upon, especially not by cooking it. Raw-foodists take all their nourishment from raw, fresh, natural foods—unadulterated by cooking.

*　　　*　　　*　　　*　　　*

Q: Why raw foods only? What's wrong with cooked foods?

A: Because cooked food is part and parcel to civilization, we have been trained never to question it. What constitutes the basis of human nourishment? Is it canned and boxed food coming out of the roaring jaws of factories? Is it the flesh of animals being churned out by factory farms? Is it the milk of cows, which is intended for baby calves? Is it cooked and processed food? The basis of human nourishment is obvious: it is RAW PLANT FOOD, which is presented to us in abundance in nature. Cooked food is adulterated and fractured, depleted of enzymes, vitamins and minerals, and starchy and clogging to the body.

*   *   *   *   *

Q: How did you come to this idea? Was it more a philosophical insight or something you learned from the scientific knowledge about health and the human body?

A: Along with David Wolfe and R.C. Dini, I came to this conclusion by pure logic. Would fire and intense heat improve one's house if applied? No, it would destroy it. And that's exactly what happens when your food is cooked, it becomes something less than it was before.

*   *   *   *   *

Q: How long have you been eating only raw foods?

A: I've been doing raw foods since 1994. With the passage of time, the distinctions become clearer and clearer and life gets better and better.

*   *   *   *   *

Q: Is there a philosophy, spirituality, or ethics behind raw-foodism, or is it just about health benefits?

A: Raw-foodism impacts every aspect of your life: mental, emotional, spiritual, and physical. So while health benefits may be what prompts a person to raw-foodism, once they adhere to it, they begin seeing the ecological and ethical impact and realizing and appreciating the spiritual benefits.

*   *   *   *   *

Q: Have you changed other areas of your life as radically?

A: The change to raw foods was not that radical. Raw foods are our natural foods. Captain Crunch is radical; cotton candy is radical; hot dogs are radical. Raw plant foods are common sense.

*   *   *   *   *

Q: What is the main reason to adopt a raw-food diet?

A: Because you want to, because you enjoy it. I can't stress this enough. I have seen so many people adopt a raw-foods lifestyle for the wrong reasons, and these people invariably fail and actually hinder their personal advancement and potential. I've seen people do it because "it's healthy," and they agonize over eating their salad while they really want to be eating a bowl of beans and rice. Yet they keep choking down the raw foods because "it's healthy." They are ingesting a lot of bad energy and cannot be truly happy or liberated, or healthy for that matter, even though that's their outward or surface reason for doing it. I've seen people do it because it seems elitist. These are the type that look down on anyone who is "not enlightened" and make others feel bad and uncomfortable, rather than sharing wanted information. These people usually lose a lot of friends and alienate their families. They also cannot be truly happy or liberated. There is nothing elitist about

The Raw-Food Diet, it is just a diet and lifestyle choice. Again, the main reason, the ONLY reason, to adopt The Raw-Food Diet is because you want to, because you enjoy it.

*   *   *   *   *

Q: What have been the most positive health benefits raw-foodism has brought to you? What do other raw-foodists say?

A: Feeling vibrant and alive is the benefit that first comes to mind for most raw-foodists, myself included.
    A feeling of well-being and healthfulness.
    Living with more clarity and consciousness
    Improved senses are another important benefit: improved eyesight, sense of smell, hearing, a clean taste palate, increased touch sensation. An improved sixth sense, intuition, is also part of that.
    The list could go on and on.

*   *   *   *   *

Q: At what point did you attain what you refer to as "Paradise Health?" After years of raw-foodism? Months? Days?

A: It's definitely not an overnight transformation, although you can start to see results immediately. You wouldn't expect to be in perfect physical shape by working out once. And the same is true with anything for that matter. Fundamentals practiced daily and consistently produce the desired results. It keeps getting better and better for me, so it's a journey that I'm still experiencing and enjoying every day.

Q: What sort of detoxification effects does the average person experience when they start adopting a raw-food diet?

A: It really depends on how you lived your life before. Someone who abused his or her body with deleterious substances is obviously going to have a heavier detoxification than someone who lived more healthfully. When the body buried in unprocessed residues of cooked food and/or other substances finally has the energy to release them, it will. There is no magic pill, only a magic process. As we untangle ourselves from cooked food, we'll release suppressed toxins and emotions. You are a work of art in progress. Each meal is a cloud or a tree or a flower, a piece of the painting that you are becoming. Every bite of food you put in your body should be adding to your perfection, to your beauty. "You are what you eat" is a cosmic law. It is known in every culture and every civilization throughout history. Every person knows that saying. Give your body the highest quality food possible.

*   *   *   *   *

Q: What do you see as the biggest challenge a raw foodist must deal with in everyday life?

A: Dealing with the rules, regulations, traditions, customs, and red tape of a dead society. It drives me crazy! People think they are free but they are not. Try walking down the street the way you came into the world (nude) and see what happens, see if you're really free. Eating raw foods at least liberates you and allows you to step outside of the current global consciousness and see what is really going on.

Q: What other lifestyle changes do you espouse besides adopting a raw food diet?

A: Eating only organic and wild foods. The commercial food of civilization is unfit for consumption and transforms people into mutants. Yes, that's harsh, but reality is harsh. When's the last time you saw a serial killer shopping at an organic produce market? Pesticides and genetically-modified food are not acceptable for the true health seeker. Humanity cannot improve upon natural foods with poisons and laboratory experiments. I also advocate abstinence from schools and universities. Modern education is an indoctrination program for the development of mediocrity and set up for the lowest common denominator. I didn't become an intelligent, successful person until I quit going to college.

*   *   *   *   *

Q: What are some more factors in overall health besides diet?

A: Along with nutrition, people must make certain the other requirements of the body are met. These include: cleanliness, exercise, rest, clean air, deep breathing, sunshine on the skin, air bathing, stretching, massage (being touched by others), intelligent thinking, loving relationships, interactions with animals, and abstinence from artificial heating and cooling. I mention cleanliness first because I feel that a lot of people that get into The Raw-Food Diet start to move away from civilized living—and that's great, to a point. It's important to untangle oneself from the mess of contemporary culture, but when one scoffs at personal hygiene and cleanliness because it's "not natural" or "cooked" to bathe, it's not healthy for them or the raw-food movement in general. It really boils my blood when I see someone that is supposed to be setting an example, trying to be a "picture of health," but they stink of body odor and have nasty, dirty hair, or an unkempt, grubby beard. The skin is the largest eliminative organ of the body. Toxins and impurities are pushed to the surface of the skin and need to be washed off. I can tell you right now that if you are living or working anywhere near automobiles, factories, cities, roads, highways, or neighborhoods, you need to be bathing every day. Your outside appearance is a reflection of your internal health. One cannot be truly healthy if one is filthy. In addition, always use a shower filter. You either filter out what is coming onto and into your body, or you become a filter.

*　　*　　*　　*　　*

Q; Have you ever encountered hostility from others when you discuss raw foods?

A: Sure, but mostly I've encountered positivity and open ears. Some people have a hard time when their belief system is challenged. Because talking about raw foods is part of my business, my work, I seldom talk about it in my personal life. I see people get into trouble when that's all they ever talk about, or they cram it down people's throats, or they make others feel uncomfortable around them because they are so judgmental. Anyone like that is a boor and a bore. As with anything, what you have to say about raw foods will fall on deaf ears unless the recipient is truly interested, unless they have initiated the conversation. I don't try to convince anyone of anything, but share information when it's wanted.

*　　*　　*　　*　　*

Q: What do you eat when you go to a restaurant or go to someone's house for dinner?

A: Almost every restaurant serves a salad, and some are even pretty good. When you go to someone's house for dinner and you do not think there will be much or anything for you to eat there, offer to bring a fruit or vegetable salad, or fruit or vegetable plate.

*   *   *   *   *

Q: Do you carry your own food everywhere?

A: When I travel, yes, I take some food with me. Airplane food is definitely not an option! I have traveled all over the world and have never had any trouble finding good food. Sometimes I hear people complain about not having raw, organic food in their area; chances are they're simply not looking hard enough.

*   *   *   *   *

Q: Do you ever eat beans or grains?

A: Beans and grains are not part of the diet I promote. They are difficult to eat raw and they are not so pleasing to the palate. They are also hard on the digestive system. There are many other better choices. For protein, green-leafy vegetables are by far the best choice. Filling and grounding foods include avocados, olives, coconuts, durians, seeds, and nuts.

*   *   *   *   *

Q: Is wheatgrass really a natural thing for humans to eat? Don't you have to grind it up in a machine to make its nutritional value accessible?

A: True, wheatgrass is not the most natural food for us, but I believe in its healing and cleansing properties and I think it is a vital part of the transition and detoxification process.

*   *   *   *   *

Q: Where is the practice of raw-foodism strongest in your opinion?

A: California.

*   *   *   *   *

Q: Do you think it's relevant to have a scientific basis to promote your idea?

A: "Science" is a tricky thing because you can prove almost anything with scientific studies, yet there will always be contradictory information from other scientific studies. That is why I am more inclined to use common sense and instinct. There have been a lot of recent studies showing the benefits of raw-foods, and I think as time goes by, raw-foodism will be normalized the way vegetarianism and veganism are now.

*   *   *   *   *

Q: What do you think of medicine, or better, of doctors as professionals in health. How often do you see one?

A: Medical doctors are coming around and some are even beginning to support The Raw-Food Diet. There is obviously a place in our modern society for doctors and western medicine. (I went to a doctor/hospital when I was in a serious car accident and would go for any kind of life-threatening emergency like that.) But the way the medical community is set up right now is disappointing: doctors having very little education on nutrition and holistic practices, patients not taking responsibility for their own health, an over-subscribing of pharmaceutical drugs, etc.

*　　　*　　　*　　　*　　　*

Q: What do you think of drugs and medicines? Why do so many people use them?

A: Drugs and medicines are toxic substances, and I can think of few cases where their benefits outweigh their ill effects. People use them because they are looking for a "magic pill" instead of taking their health into their own hands, and because drugs and medicines are over-prescribed by doctors. Most people don't know any better, and just blindly follow their doctor's orders, and most doctors are trained to treat illnesses and pathologies with drugs.

*　　　*　　　*　　　*　　　*

Q: Do you take any nutritional supplements?

A: Yes, I take superfoods and supplements now. At first, I was really into the 100% raw purist thing, then I learned more about the really high-quality superfoods/supplements out there, and I'm glad I did. One can still develop deficiencies even on a vegan raw-food diet. You can't just eat sweet fruit all day and expect your optimal nutritional needs to be met. All the really successful, super-healthy, long-term raw-foodists I know eat a balanced raw-food diet consisting of organic, mineral-dense fruits, vegetables, nuts, seeds, superfoods, and raw supplements. The best superfoods and supplements I have found over the years are: Nature's First Food (an all-raw, all-organic green superfood/probiotic blend), Liver Rescue (an all-raw milk-thistle/dandelion/artichoke extract that supports optimal liver function), Beauty Antioxidant (the broadest spectrum of pyc-nogenols and other highly potent anti-aging antioxidants known), Tocotrienols (a raw superfood form of vitamin E), Pure Radiance C (the top vitamin C in the world made from Camu Camu berries), Nature's First Law Bee Pollen (collected from the rainforests of New Zealand), and Vita Synergy (the most amazing and nutritionally-dense multi-vitamin available in the world, including over 3000% of the RDA of vitamin B12, which is great for vegans!).

* * * * *

Q: Aren't humans omnivorous, meaning that we can eat from both the animal and plant kingdoms? Haven't our bodies evolved to digest almost everything; our teeth and mouth, mus-cles and enzymes being adapted to this kind of nutrition? Aren't we ignoring, and maybe contradicting all this when we refuse to eat meat, even raw meat?

A: Just because we are able to chew something up and excrete it does not mean that we are biologically designed to eat that food. If I am able to eat cotton candy, does that mean that I'm an omnivore? No, cotton candy is terrible for me and I am going to pay the price for eating it. Every degeneration in our food leads to a subsequent degeneration in our bodies.

* * * * *

Q: What do you think is one of the biggest problems ailing modern society?

A: Addiction. Addiction to being in a toxic physiological con-dition actually. People are constantly trying to reach a level of euphoria artificially, which is theirs naturally.

Q: You say that, "food-combining principles were formulated by and for cooked-food eaters, they don't pertain to you." This sounds very much like some statements in T.C. Fry's Healthful Living Newsletter, saying that food-combining was for the biologically compromised (sick) and not always necessary for persons of robust health. Since many of the recipes in your book combine fruits, nuts, and vegetables in a blender and so forth, might you elaborate upon this for the readers?

A: Food combining rules are for people with poor absorption and poor digestion and are not always necessary for healthy people. My cycles change and my diet changes, and I eat in "strange" combinations now, but that's what makes me feel great. The combinations that work for me may not necessarily work for others, and vice versa.

*   *   *   *   *

Q: I notice that you advocate colon irrigations. To many natural hygienists it was a blessing to be free of such dogma to simply allow their bodies to heal through "intelligently doing nothing." Why direct your readers to this non-hygienic Dr. Ehret-esque "mucusless" mentality?

A: In some cases, there are residues in the body (gall stones, impacted fecal matter, etc.) that are "stuck." As with the amalgam fillings people want removed from their mouths, intestinal residue removal may have to be assisted mechanically. Decades of eating fragmented, clogging foods can't always be eliminated by the body through proper eating.

*   *   *   *   *

Q: Can a raw foodist overdose on a particular food? For example, could someone eat too much of one food?

A: Yes, definitely. In my partner David Wolfe's book, "The Sunfood Diet Success System," he explains how to keep oneself balanced on raw foods. In my opinion, David's "Sunfood Triangle" is really a landmark dietary distinction. The Triangle consists of the three essentials to The Raw-Food Diet: Greens, Sugars, and Fats. These foods balance against each other and keep you centered. He also describes the symptoms of food overdoses (the symptoms of eating too much fruit sugar, too many greens, etc.)

It's different for everyone. Someone may be able to eat only cherries for a week when they first come in season, and they may feel great. While another person couldn't eat just cherries for one day without feeling unbalanced. Each person needs to find their own balance.

                *   *   *   *   *

Q: On a raw foods diet you are putting a very high quality "fuel" into your system. It seems as though it is easy to spend a lot of money quickly eating a totally raw organic diet. Any advice for someone having trouble dishing out the extra cash?

A: I keep the costs low by eating what is in season. Obviously, eating something like cherries in the winter is going to be expensive because cherries' harvest season is summer. Also, eating what is in season is Nature's way of telling you what to eat. (Note: For these reasons, I included the Seasonal Produce Availability section in this book which lists the peak seasons for all fruits and vegetables.) Another thing to consider is to never penny-pinch when it comes to your health. You can penny-pinch somewhere else in your budget, but definitely not in your health and diet. People who aren't willing to pay for the highest-quality foods now are going to get less than excellent results in their health and vitality—and those results could end up with visits to a doctor or hospital, which will be much more expensive than organic produce.

*   *   *   *   *

Q: A lot of people's first reaction to a raw foods diet is "I could never do that..." or "I just couldn't give up..." What would you say to these people?

A: I'd say, "Yes, you will be giving up many dead and poisoned foods that are unhealthy and doing your body and soul an extreme disservice. You will be stepping outside your comfort zone and experiencing something totally new and amazing. You will experience for the first time in your life feelings of well-being, vibrancy, and euphoria far better than any drug high. Your newly-found taste buds will wake up from their numbness and experience hundreds of new fresh, high-quality, delicious foods. You will meet hundreds, if not thousands, of amazing people on your journey—people who are not a part of the herd (which is plundering into the abyss); people who are part of the solution, not part of the problem; people with insights, stories, and lessons that exceed those of even the greatest philosophers, movie-makers, and university professors. You will look back on your old life and see that your comfort zone was never comfortable at all."

*   *   *   *   *

Q: Is The Raw-Food Diet for everyone?

A: No, The Raw-Food Diet is for people with a success-consciousness—a strong desire to better themselves physically, mentally, and spiritually. The Raw-Food Diet is for people who wish to advance toward their full potential. It's a shame that the vast majority of people on this planet have little or no concern for these things.

*   *   *   *   *

Part II: Weight Training & Bodybuilding

*   *   *   *   *

Q: Your Raw Power! Program is said to be the only program about building strength and muscles naturally (raw). What is the general idea behind it?

A: My program is about how to have the exact body that you've always desired—a beautifully fit, strong, healthy, and vibrant body. Now, many people already know that a raw-food diet is the natural way to eat, but some people have difficulty building strength and gaining healthy muscular weight. The Raw Power! Program is about attaining a high level of health, eating a 100% natural diet, true natural body-building, and total fitness. The only way to build your body naturally is through eating naturally.

*   *   *   *   *

Q: What is your concept of bodybuilding, and how does it differ from similar activities, such as weight training for conditioning, powerlifting, and Olympic-style weightlifting?

A: My concept of bodybuilding is building and maintaining a super-strong and super-healthy body, free from illness and disease. My program combines natural body-building, weight-lifting, total fitness, conditioning, and diet information that is specifically designed for building and maintaining muscle and strength.

Q: Does your program appeal to body-builders only?

A: My program appeals to anyone with a desire to better themselves mentally and physically. All the other books on diet and fitness, or diet and body-building, are erroneous. Cooked food does not build a body; cooked food destroys a body in the long run. Raw Power! appeals to everybody, whether you want to look like a raw version of Arnold Schwarzenegger, or you just want a slim, muscular body capable of endless energy and stamina.

*   *   *   *   *

Q: How many people have you trained in conventional body-building, and how many people have you trained all raw?

A: Many of both. I receive hundreds of calls and emails every day, so a lot of what I do now is consulting. I used to train more people in the gym, but I currently concentrate mostly on seminars and consulting.

*   *   *   *   *

Q: For all-raw training, what is the difference between training someone who is already experienced at conventional body-building versus training someone who has no prior bodybuilding experience? Who is easier or better to train as far as success?

A: It's really an individual thing. The people that make building strength and muscle naturally their number one priority are always the most fun to train. I love seeing and meeting people that are my equal as far as dedication and motivation; it pushes me closer to my full potential. A person can either have "champion mentality" or "spectator mentality," the choice is theirs. It's the people that want something for nothing that are difficult to train and deal with.

*   *   *   *   *

Q: Why do most raw-foodists seem to have problems keeping up their strength and weight?

A: Well, first and foremost, a lot of people that get into the raw-food diet seem to come from a life of sickness and hypochondriacal behavior. So, with that type of mentality, it's only natural that they fail at achieving their goal health and physique. People must conclusively decide that they want to gain strength and weight and make it their number one priority. People want a quick fix, they want to gain weight and muscle now, today, yesterday! Harnessing the power of mind is key. If you truly know in your mind that you can accomplish a goal, you can do it. I believe in The Self-Fulfilling Prophecy, if you think you can't build strength and muscle, then you can't.

*   *   *   *   *

Q: How does exercise play into your life, and how are your strength and physical capabilities affected by raw-foodism? Can one expect the same results from weight training and cardiovascular exercise on the raw-food diet as one can from such exercise while eating cooked food?

A: I am very big into weight-training. I hit the weights about 5 days a week and walk, hike, or run every day. You have to detoxify all the toxic waste and poisons out of your body (experience the weight loss and occasional weakness) before you can build up on raw foods. You have to be willing to detoxify all the way. From my experience on a raw-food diet, it is easily

possible to gain muscle and unleash strength that you never
knew you had.

*   *   *   *   *

Q: How do recovery rates and the need for sleep and rest differ between conventional bodybuilders and all-raw bodybuilders?

A: Conventional bodybuilders eat all day (5 or 6 big meals
plus shakes and snacks) and run their metabolism at an accel-
erated rate; thus they recover slower and need more sleep
because the body is constantly expending energy digesting,
assimilating, and eliminating foods.   All-raw bodybuilders
recover faster if they include significant amounts of green-leafy
vegetable juice (16-24 ounces) into their daily diet regime.

*   *   *   *   *

Q: How do raw foods affect athletic performance?

A: The raw-foodist athlete has an immeasurable advantage.
Building a body with cooked-food nutrition is similar to blow-
ing up a balloon; sooner or later the balloon will deflate.
Muscles "blown up" with cooked food and other unnatural substances will eventually atrophy and "deflate." Most fitness
experts and bodybuilders atrophy and wear down prematurely.
Muscles built on raw-food nutrition last much longer because
they are built naturally. I compare building your body with
cooked food to building a house without any foundation.
Sooner or later, that house is going to crumble.

Q: Do you think a raw food bodybuilder could ever compete against steroid takers in the strength and girth departments?

A: Definitely so.   If you think about it logically, all the largest and strongest mammals on Earth are 100% raw plant eaters. The gorilla, the elephant, the hippopotamus, the giraffe, the rhinoceros, the horse, the bull, the buffalo, and so on, are all 100% raw plant eaters! A gorilla has the strength equivalent to bench-pressing 4,000 pounds. What rule of science says that a gorilla is able to synthesize proteins from raw plant foods but we are not? There are no raw food bodybuilders competing against steroid takers in the strength and girth departments because people simply are not aware of the potential of building strength and muscle naturally on The Raw-Food Diet.

*   *   *   *   *

Q: You seem to naturally be a pretty big guy, but have you ever successfully trained a skinny person into being a big guy with your all raw methods? Going from skinny to big and muscular happens routinely and dramatically with conventional bodybuilding, so how about with all raw?

A: Yes, I was blessed with good genetics. I could probably eat at McDonalds every day and still live into my nineties like my grandparents.   But that's not what this is all about. Implementing the Raw Power! Bodybuilding Method is about adding life to your years, as well as years to your life. Yes, I train and consult skinny people every day. Those that are dedicated always have tremendous results. Presently, I have been training David Wolfe. In the past year and a half he has gained 15 pounds of lean muscle. He discusses his experiences in his book **The Sunfood Diet Success System.**

Q: What do you think your potential would be if you did conventional bodybuilding?

A: The potential of anyone eating unnaturally is a short term gain at the expense of a long term tragedy. Sure, you can build huge muscles eating meat and injecting steroids and guzzling pills and protein powders, but there is a tremendous price to pay in the end.

*   *   *   *   *

Q: Are you personally stronger now than when you were a cooked-food eater?

A: I can say that I'm at least twice as strong now as I was when I was eating a Standard American Diet. I used to bench-press 300 pounds three times, now I can bench that weight twenty times. That's a huge improvement in brute strength. On a burnout set, I used to benchpress 135 pounds forty times, now I can bench that weight well over one hundred times. That's a huge improvement in muscular endurance. I also find that I need little or no rest between sets of exercises now.

*   *   *   *   *

Q: What are your current "vital statistics." Besides your height and weight, which you've already divulged, would you also reveal your body fat percentage, blood pressure, and heart rate, as well as the girth measurements of your neck, shoulders, chest, arms, forearms, wrist, waist, hips, thighs, calves, and ankles?

A: I'm not into all that; the only measurement for me is how vibrant I feel. I used to measure my arms when I was younger, but I realize now that measurements prove very little. Though its arms aren't very big, a chimpanzee can rip a car door off of its hinges. I've seen "bodybuilders" with 22-inch arms that can't benchpress 300 pounds. I'm going for chimpanzee strength, not big measurements.

* * * * *

Q: Do you recommend maximum lifts? Why or why not?

A: I don't do maximum lifts anymore. This is because I prefer to train alone. It's obviously not wise to do maximum lifts without a training partner or spot. Training alone has its downfalls for some people, but, at this point in my life, I cannot tolerate a gym atmosphere (cooked/meat-eater sweat and smells, air conditioning, terrible music, crowded, etc.). Another interesting thing to note is that when I used to go to the gym, as soon as someone found out that I don't eat cooked food, meat, pills, or steroids, I would become an attraction. People would watch me work out, which I hate. I would end up talking about The Raw-Food Diet and my workouts would suffer. If you have a quality training partner and are in great shape, I see no reason why you couldn't perform maximum lifts.

* * * * *

Q: What are your reasons for bodybuilding? Is it because you are vain and ego-centric, as some critics accuse bodybuilders of being? I mean, why do it? Why not just relax and stay skinny? Since lot of people think that bodybuilding is a waste of time and energy, what would you say to convince someone that they should body build?

A: I like feeling strong, and I like the feeling of being pumped up. I don't try to convince anyone of anything. I'm just presenting information showing that one can gain weight and muscle on a raw-food diet and without undermining one's health with unnatural nutrition.

*   *   *   *   *

Q: Don't you have a reason beyond feeling strong and pumped as motivation to lift weights?

A: Arnold Schwarzenegger once said that being pumped up feels better than an orgasm! I don't know if I would go that far, but he has a good point! Being pumped up feels great, and I have yet to be in a bad mood after a good workout. That's my motivation for lifting weights, to feel great.

*   *   *   *   *

Q: Why do some raw-food eaters seem to be lacking the "definition" and "vascularity" that most raw food eaters or even cooked food bodybuilders have?

A: I have long thought that definition is not always healthy (concentration camp prisoners all had definition!). In my opinion, the massive, defined, ripped, professional bodybuilders of today have accepted the ultimate Faustian bargain. They fill their bodies with absurd nutritional pollution just to look "defined." Then they wonder why they have completely broken down (or died) by the time they are "middle-aged." Muscle definition has a lot to do with genetics and body type. My brother and I have worked out with weights just about every day for the last 15 years (I'm talking hard-core workouts), and we are very strong, but with very little definition. So, it's a mystery to me as well, but I don't worry about it. Nature determines your natural body type. Think of your health first and foremost, the definition will either be there or not. The race for the lowest body-fat percentage is a kamikaze crash-course.

Q: Many animals do show vascularity and muscle striations in their natural state. Mightn't we also? I used to think definition was genetic, too, until I was all raw and finally saw all of my abdominal muscles in clear awesome cuts. Might not diet be the deciding factor on definition and vascularity?

A: Well, I have found that my definition was "best" about 7 years ago, when I was eating a high protein diet (meat, eggs, milk, etc.). But now that I'm raw, I'm much stronger and I feel much better. That's all I really care about. If I can't see all my abdominal muscles in clear awesome cuts, I don't care as long as I feel great. And you're correct, many animals do show vascularity and muscle striations in their natural state, and many animals do not, yet they are very strong and powerful.

*   *   *   *   *

Q: Where do you get enough protein for real muscle growth?

A: Where does a cow, rhinoceros, hippopotamus, or gorilla get enough protein for real muscle development and growth? Raw plant foods. Protein synthesis is protein synthesis.

*   *   *   *   *

Q: I have heard it takes about a year to build ten pounds of muscle tissue. Do you feel that the ten to fifteen pound range is about the maximum growth curve that a raw body builder has?

A: I don't ever put limitations on anything. If someone wanted to gain, say, 20 pounds of muscle in a year, it could be done. It fully depends on the conviction, persistence, and determination of the individual.

Q: Would you explain why coconut and avocado are necessary for you and whether there may be another way to gain weight if one doesn't want to, or can't go, the coconut and avocado route?

A: Fat is the delivery device to the muscles and bones of minerals drawn from green-leafed vegetables. One could use coconuts, avocados, olives, or nuts. I personally enjoy all four. Olives are one of the best foods for bodybuilding.

*   *   *   *   *

Q: How can one gain more weight on one or two large meals, as you recommend, rather than on many small meals throughout the day?

A: This slows down the metabolism, allowing one to more easily gain weight. It is very simple and demonstrable to anyone who tries it.

*   *   *   *   *

Q: You mention fasting once a week, yet some would say that it is unnecessary or even harmful to fast this often if one is already eating a biologically correct diet. Would you explain the reasoning behind your fasts?

A: Again, this slows the metabolism. The digestive organs need an occasional rest. The whole body does.

*   *   *   *   *

Q: How often do you work out?

A: Five times a week on average. I'd like to work out more,

but I have many obligations right now—a family, a homestead, and a fast-growing business.

* * * * *

Q: Do you find that the raw food diet tends to make high-rep training more the way to go rather than high-poundage training?

A: Combining the two would be optimal. High-reps with high-poundage!

* * * * *

Q: You stated that one should train in the sun whenever possible. This is a refreshing change from the solar phobia of skin cancer warnings that we hear these days. What are the benefits of training in the sun?

A: Increased blood flow in the muscles, increase testosterone levels, fresher air, and the opening up of stagnated, contracted areas of the body.

* * * * *

Q: You mention that sexual abstinence is desirable to help conserve body nutrients before exercise or competition. Isn't this just an old wives tale perpetuated by trainers to keep their athletes away form the distraction of a new romance?

A: No, it definitely is a reality. If one is constantly draining one's sexual energy, it makes strength gains very difficult. Two closely matched training partners that have the difference of one being sexually active and one not will notice the strength difference. This is not to imply complete sexual abstinence, but abstinence before work-outs.

*   *   *   *   *

Q: Do you ever take layoffs?

A: Yes, when I go on trips. It is good to give your body a rest once in a while so when you come back, you are fresh and motivated.

*   *   *   *   *

Q: You use free weights, right? Why do you prefer them?

A: Free weights allow for a free range of motion, and they require the individual to use her/his own balance. I have found that when I concentrate on mechanics (form), I get a much better workout.

*   *   *   *   *

Q: Do you use any aerobics in your training?

A: Yes, running, hiking, and swimming.

*   *   *   *   *

Q: What should a very young all raw bodybuilder know regarding his special considerations?

A: Start where you are. Build up slowly.

Q: Is your program useful to the advanced bodybuilder?

A: Definitely. Before now, I doubt the advanced bodybuilder has ever come across information that says that one can be super-strong without wearing one's body down prematurely with pills and cooked foods.

*   *   *   *   *

Q: Do you plan to write a book strictly for the hard core advanced and/or competition bodybuilders?

A: Raw Power! is all anyone needs. The Men's Advanced Workout is tough! I challenge any hard-core bodybuilder to follow it for 3 months. Most hard-core bodybuilders are too cooked and don't have the stamina; they can't complete the whole workout.

*   *   *   *   *

Q: How much time do you think should someone devote to taking care of his/her body?

A: I take good care of myself 24 hours a day, 7 days a week. Anything less than that is harmful to one's well-being.

*   *   *   *   *

Part III – Nature's First Law

*   *   *   *   *

Q: What is Nature's First Law?

A: Nature's First Law is the business my partner David Wolfe and I started in 1994. We are an internet and mail order business and we also have a retail store in San Diego, California. We distribute "resources for massive health abundance," books, audio and video tapes, juicers, dehydrators, water filters, dried organic fruits, organic nuts and seeds, organic olives and olive oil, superfoods, and many more raw lifestyle products. We sell the items we use in our own lives, items we know other people want to buy and use too. Our catalog and inventory grow larger all the time as we add more select products. We also host raw-food events, health retreats and seminars all over the world. "Nature's First Law: The Raw Food Diet" is a book that David Wolfe, R.C. Dini and I wrote. It is already on its fifth edition and is becoming increasingly popular.

*   *   *   *   *

Q: Your organization, Nature's First Law, has been called the "militant wing" of the raw-food movement.

A: Yes, I guess we come across as uncompromising, and we do so purposefully. When we wrote "Nature's First Law: The Raw Food Diet," we knew we wanted to shake things up, shake people up. We wanted to provoke action. I like absolutist writing and we wanted the book to be a manifesto of sorts. Our critics say the book and our style are alienating, that they turn people off. All I have to do is think about all of the people our book and our style have turned ON! Our rhetoric is very powerful... sometimes we overdo it. No, our book is not for everyone. Nothing is for everyone. But you'd be surprised by the diverse people we do appeal to, by the many, many lives we've touched and changed. And that's what I care about, not being likeable or popular.

Q: Do you think we have any "duty" to live as Nature intended, or is it just something we can do if we personally value Nature?

A: We at Nature's First Law feel it is our moral and ethical obligation to live consciously and conscientiously. What we eat deeply and radically affects how we think, feel, and behave, it directly affects how we interact with the planet. In that sense, it is a duty. Switching to a raw-food diet has a massive positive impact on the environment as well as ourselves. Life change comes from the inside out. Once you change on the inside, everything changes on the outside.

*   *   *   *   *

Q: What are the current changes and trends in the raw-foods movement?

A: Information sharing. The Internet has really done a great service for the world by making basically any information on any subject available to anyone with computer access. The Raw Food Movement has benefited greatly from this technology as well. Anyone interested in starting or maintaining a raw-food diet can access my Internet website at, you guessed it, www.rawfood.com—this website is the largest resource of information, products, and organic food for this diet and lifestyle. The internet is the vehicle for so many of the things our company is doing. We use our website to connect people. We have a Premier Raw-Foodists page, which gives bios and contact information on those "who have gone before." We have a board for discussions and information sharing. We have a site for singles ads for people to connect with others with similar values. One of our most popular features is our email bulletin, which keeps people up-to-date on new products, happenings in

the raw-food world, and events worldwide. (If you would like
to sign up for this email bulletin, email nature@rawfood.com)

We feel strongly about putting a lot back into the raw-food
community. We have spent years networking, meeting other
raw-foodists around the world, reviewing and adding new products to our catalog, and connecting people in order to make the
raw-food community successful and welcoming to new-comers.

*   *   *   *   *

**Additional questions may be answered
by Stephen Arlin online at:
stephen@rawfood.com**

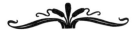

The Ultimate Raw Bodybuilding Sample Menu Plan

People frequently ask me what I eat from the beginning of the day to the end. Well, it's always different, but there are some things that I eat and drink on a consistent basis: olives, greens, avocados, coconuts, distilled water, green juice, and Nature's First Food superfood. Following is a sample menu plan that works great for me. Try it out and fine-tune it to fit your personal needs:

7:00am: 24-oz. distilled water with lemon juice, two Liver Rescue caps, two Pure Radiance C caps, three Vita Synergy tablets

8:00am: Light Workout (walking, running, hiking, swimming, yoga, etc.)

9:45am: Two Beauty Antioxidant chewable caps

10:00am: Super-smoothie (one tablespoon of Nature's First Food superfood, one tablespoon Tocotrienols, one tablespoon NFL Bee Pollen, one handful goji berries, and the juice of one young coconut)

12:00pm: Huge dark-green salad with "Raw Power Olives," avocados, cabbage, cucumbers, hemp seeds, and homemade raw salad dressing

3:00pm: Macadamia nuts, goji berries, and romaine lettuce leaves

4:00pm: Heavy Workout (weight-training)

6:00pm: Huge dark-green salad with "Raw Power Olives," avocados, cabbage, cucumbers, hemp seeds, and homemade raw salad dressing

8:00pm: Super-smoothie (one tablespoon of Nature's First Food superfood, one tablespoon Tocotrienols, one tablespoon NFL Bee Pollen, one handful goji berries, and the juice of one young coconut)

8:45pm: snack (pumpkin seed butter on flaxseed crackers)

9:00pm: Submission Fighting Training (martial arts)

11:00pm: 24-oz. distilled water with lemon juice, two Liver Rescue caps, two Pure Radiance C caps

Try this menu plan (and variations of it) for 60 days. You should make substitutions to keep the diet interesting. For example, you can substitute zucchini for cucumbers, or pecans for macadamia nuts, etc. There are also many phenomenal recipes to choose from in the next section.

Raw Power! Recipes
by Jolie

One's success on the raw-food diet
hinges on one's salad dressing.
— Susan Kosich

TO EAT RAW RECIPES
(aka "combo abombos")
OR NOT

There are many schools of thought on how to eat a raw-food diet. Some say you should eat only foods in their whole, unprocessed state. Some say you should eat a mono diet, meaning only one food at a time. Some say the typical raw-food recipe does not follow optimal food-combining principles and can be difficult to digest. They are all correct to some degree. It may be optimal to eat a mono-diet of whole foods. And if that is the diet you enjoy and it makes you feel the best, then read no further. But for a lot of people, the flavor, creativity and variety that raw-food recipes offer make all the difference in eating an all-raw or predominantly raw-food diet, as opposed to falling back into old, tastier habits. As the above quote implies, if a great salad dressing means that you eat more greens, then hurray! If raw-food recipes make your lunches fun and your dinners something to look forward to, hip-hip-hurray!

Everyone's dietary needs (and tastes for that matter) are different. And everyone's dietary needs change as they go through different stages of life. Not only is there no one way for everyone to eat, there is no one way for one person to eat.

For example, eating simple mono meals may be the best diet for a person who is cleansing or simplifying their life. Several months later, eating big salads and tasty recipes may be just what that person needs to feel nourished and happy. We simply have to approach this subject with intelligence, intuition, and a light heart. Be happy and trust in yourself. Don't become too serious about food. You are your own best expert and you will know how to fine-tune your diet.

ABOUT THE RECIPES

Stephen and I have chosen a variety of recipes that support body-building. They are relatively easy to make, with the exceptions requiring a time investment that is well worth it.

The Vegetable Dips & Salad Dressings section has been expanded since we think knowing how to make good dips and dressings is important and can make all the difference in enjoying and feeling satiated from one's raw-food meals.

Stephen has also included some of the recipes from Raw Power! first edition at the end of the section.

ABOUT THE INGREDIENTS

Use organic ingredients whenever possible. Use purified or revitalised distilled water. Adhering to these and the following practices will make your recipes taste absolutely fresh, nutritious and delicious!

HERBS AND SPICES

Use fresh, organic or wild-crafted herbs when possible.

De-stem your fresh herbs before using in recipes. I use dried herbs during the winter or when fresh are not available. I either dry them myself or I acquire dried herbs from our local food co-op. If you purchase dried herbs, make sure they are organic or wild-crafted and that they have not been irradiated. Usually the type you can get in the bulk section of your food co-op or health food store is your best bet. Take note that dried herbs give a recipe a flavor different from fresh.

The class of food condiments labeled "Spices" includes all kinds of things, from seeds (cumin, cardamom, fennel seed), to roots (ginger, turmeric, fennel root), to chiles and peppers, and more. I try to prepare most of my spices myself using whichever method is most appropriate for the job: seed grinder, mortar and pestle, kitchen scissors, etc. Sometimes you can find organic or wild-crafted spices that have not been irradiated. Ask lots of questions about how the spices are processed. Again, your best bet is the spice bulk section of your food co-op or health food store.

SALT

I use Celtic sea salt in my recipes. Regular table salt is definitely out as it has been treated with chemicals and irradiated. There are those who object to any salt consumption, regardless of the source (especially natural hygienists). It is true that salt can cause edema and retarded digestion if it is over-consumed. I think it is fine to abstain from all salt or to consume small amounts of it, whichever fits your physiology and your tastes. If you are used to abstaining from salt, my recipes will taste fine without it. Otherwise, I usually give a range (for example, 1-3 teaspoons salt), and you should always start on the low end, adding more if need be. You can always add more salt but you can't take it out.

NAMA SHOYU

Nama Shoyu is an unpasteurized, organic soy sauce known as "The Champagne of Soy Sauces." It is touted for being enzyme-rich and lower in salt than traditional soy sauce. It is used by some raw-foodists in place of Bragg's Liquid Aminos, nutritional yeast, and other salty products. The big question is, is it raw? The answer is no, but it's worth knowing more.

The ingredients are as follows: organically-grown whole soybeans, water, organically-grown whole wheat, sea salt, and aspergillus oryzae (koji). Koji is boiled organic whole wheat covered by a full bloom of the aspergillus oryzae mold. As you may know, molds are often used as agents to break down soybeans or grains into easily-digestible forms. (This type of fermentation process is a kind of predigestion.) The koji is then added to boiled organic soy beans. This is fermented in cedar vats for two years, at which time more boiled soybeans and wheat are added, then it is fermented for another two years. Cedar is well-known for being enzyme-rich and the cedar vats used by the makers of Nama Shoyu are over 150 years old. Because of the unique double-brew process, Nama Shoyu can be made with 17% less salt than common soy sauce.

The bottom line is that nutritious, enzyme-packed Nama Shoyu is really a "live food" product, not a raw-food product. It's essentially fermented cooked food.

For purists, Nama Shoyu is not really an option. But compared to Bragg's, which is 100% cooked and void of enzymes, Nama Shoyu is a great alternative. It can possibly help bridge the gap from salty cooked foods to unadulterated raw-food eating for some people. Like any food condiment, it should be used sparingly, and anyone in-tune with their body will know if they're "over doing it."

Nama Shoyu can be omitted from most of my recipes that call for it, with the exception of the recipes that include my Asian Dressing/Marinade (page 115).

MISO

Miso that is labeled "raw" or "unpasteurized" falls into the same category as Nama Shoyu. It is a fermented cooked food. It is also rich in enzymes and a nutritious, tasty, salty-food substitute. There are many different types of miso (red, dark, blonde, etc.) made from many different bases. Just make sure it is organic and unpasteurized and experiment to find your favorite. If you are new to miso, I suggest trying the lighter ones first (they will be called "blonde," "white," or "golden").

NUTS

I almost always crack my own nuts, so I buy them in-shell. Shelled nuts roll along the conveyor belt after they are shelled, then they are bagged and boxed and trucked around and warehoused until they make it to your food co-op or health food store. Then they are put into the bulk bins and sit there until you buy them. That's a lot of time and exposure for oxidizing. Of course in-shell nuts go through all of this travelling too, but in their protective little shells. In addition to being more intact, freshly-shelled nuts taste so much better than mechanically shelled nuts. (Try a side-by-side taste test to experience the difference yourself.) This is not to say that shelled nuts are void of all beneficial properties, or that it's always realistic to shell your own, it's just food for thought. One hint to make cracking macadamias easier is refrigerating them for an hour or more before cracking them. Also, the Krakanut is the best nut-cracker there is and a great help in cracking your own nuts (see description in next section, The 21st Century Kitchen).

Soaking vs. not soaking. There are many people in the raw and living-food communities that recommend soaking or sprouting all nuts and seeds before eating them or including them in recipes. This is to remove or release the nut or seed's enzyme inhibitors, which are Mother Nature's form of preservative (they preserve the nut or seed for future plant reproduction). The enzyme inhibitors are said to tax one's pancreas and other organs, deplete one's pancreatic enzymes and cause gastrointestinal problems. The trouble I have with this is that most of the information on this subject comes from animal studies (small laboratory animals being fed large quantities of enzyme inhibitors) and human studies of humans eating a mostly cooked-food diet. I personally am not convinced that it is "natural" to eat nuts or seeds in this form and I don't know that it is necessary. I also don't care as much for the taste of soaked or sprouted nuts and seeds; it's more of a sproutish taste. I adore the creamy texture of nuts and seeds, especially in my recipes. If you do decide to soak or sprout your nuts and seeds, the recipes will still work out just fine. I do sometimes soak my nuts or seeds for 15-30 minutes just to make mixing them a little easier. If you are eating a lot of nuts and seeds and they aren't agreeing with you, then try soaking to see if it works for you.

GRAINS

The reason many raw-foodists avoid grains is that they can upset one's digestive system. I have certainly experienced this in the past. I think part of the problem is that we may eat too much grain in one sitting or one day, or even one week.

Grains are very easy to over-do because the amount we should eat is probably very small.

I guess just as vegetarians and vegans are often trying to make meat substitutes, raw-foodists are often trying to make cooked grain and bread substitutes. Well, we can't eat soaked or sprouted grains in the same ways we can cooked grains. Instead of gobbling down a big bowl of grains, we have to change our thinking and just add grains in to other dishes, as almost more of a condiment (the way we sprinkle sunflower seeds over our salads). Or as a "supplement," for soaked or sprouted grains will add staying power to any meal.

Our family includes sprouted grains in our meals occasionally. It is a sustaining food, which is very important for growing children, active adults and those who feel they need something more filling in their diet. We just eat a little at a time, about 1/4 cup per person and we don't seem to have any digestive problems this way. This is what I recommend.

Because it is easier to digest, unhybridized, and so easy to work with, kamut is my first grain of choice. Other choices for variety are quinoa, millet, barley, and occasionally wild rice. It is beyond the scope of this recipe section to go into sprouting grains, but there are many raw-food recipe books that discuss the process in detail, complete with charts and all.

You almost can't go wrong with kamut. Just soak one cup of it in 4 cups of water for 24 hours. It can be drained and used then (this is when I prefer to use it), or drained and sprouted for a day or two before being used.

Wild rice (which is actually the seed of tall water grass that grows in the Great Lakes area) is also popular among raw-foodists. It never does sprout so it just needs to be soaked until it is soft and chewy, which takes from 1-5 days.

You must chew sprouted grains very well, but you'll be used to that after all the salad and veggies you've been eating!

Instead of raw pilafs and other grain dish recipes, I'll just give you some ideas:

- Add 2 T sprouted grains to a smoothie
- Add 2 T sprouted grains to your favorite blended soup
- Sprinkle sprouted grains over a salad
- Marinate 1/2 C soaked kamut or other sprouted grain in 2 T of salad dressing
- Add 2 T soaked or sprouted grains to your nut patés
- Marinate 1/2 C soaked kamut in 1/2 tsp Nama Shoyu and 1/2 tsp Omega Chili/Garlic flax oil

Note - Gluten sensitivity is a very real thing. There are many people who suffer from celiac disease and many others who suffer from non-celiac gluten sensitivity. If you know or think you suffer from gluten sensitivity, avoid kamut and barley (and miso and Nama Shoyu for that matter). You should be safe with sprouting quinoa, millet, and wild rice.

TECHNIQUE

There are a lot of techniques utilized in a raw-foods kitchen, but one in particular that I want to mention here. When you are mixing thicker recipes in your food processor or blender (nut patés, coconut custard, etc.) you may need to "coach" the mixing along. This means that you may need to mix for a moment, stop the motor, scrape down the sides of the mixing bowl with a spatula, then start again. You may also need to stop the motor and hand mix the ingredients before starting again. This may sound tedious, but it's not, and before you know it, it will be second nature. This will help you achieve the desired consistency in the food you are making.

SERVING RAW FOOD

It seems to help with a lot of raw-food dishes to take the chill off, especially in cold weather. There are actually only a few things I enjoy chilled--watermelon, smoothies, some veggie dips, that kind of thing. When served at room temperature, foods are more flavorful and easier to digest. It only takes about 15 minutes to bring something down to room temperature. If you are not going to consume all of a food, don't bring it all down to room temperature. Just take what you're going to eat and leave the rest in the refrigerator.

VEGETABLE DIPS & SALAD DRESSINGS

AVO DILL DIP

2 ripe avocados
1/2 C fresh dill
3 T fresh-squeezed orange juice
2 T fresh-squeezed lemon juice
1-2 cloves garlic
1 tsp sea salt (optional)

Scoop avocados out with a spoon. Mix all ingredients in food processor until smooth. Makes 2 cups. Best if served chilled.

AVO BASIL DIP

2 ripe avocados
1 C fresh basil
the fresh-squeezed juice from 1/2 of a lemon
1-2 cloves garlic
1 tsp sea salt

Scoop avocados out with a spoon. Mix all ingredients in food processor until smooth. Makes 2 cups. Best if served chilled.

HUZZIE'S BEST GUACAMOLE

4 avocados
1 medium tomato, diced (Roma tomatoes work best)
2 T chives, chopped
1/8 tsp red pepper flakes
1/2 tsp celtic sea salt
1/4 C pitted olives, chopped (optional)

Pit avocados and scoop into a mixing bowl. Add red pepper flakes and salt, then mash with a "potato" masher or large fork until a rich, creamy consistency is achieved. Add tomatoes, chives and olives and stir. Makes 3 1/2 to 4 cups.

CREAMY GUACAMOLE DIP

2 ripe avocados
1-2 tomatoes
1/4 C fresh cilantro
1/2 small onion
2 cloves garlic
1 tsp chopped red jalapeno pepper or other red pepper
1 T fresh-squeezed lemon juice
1 tsp sea salt

Scoop avocados out with a spoon. Mix all ingredients in food processor until smooth. Makes 2 cups. Best if served chilled. You can also make this chunky style if you prefer, chopping everything and mixing together by hand.

Variations - Use lime juice instead of lemon juice.
   - Add 1-2 T pinenuts for a deliciously unusual flavor.

RANCH DIP or DRESSING

1 1/2 C cashews or macadamias
1/2 C water
3 T fresh lemon juice
1-2 cloves garlic
1-2 tsp sea salt
1/2 tsp dried dill (or 1 very small sprig fresh)
1/2 tsp dried basil (or 2 leaves fresh)
1 stalk celery

Mix all ingredients in Vita-Mix or blender until smooth and creamy. Makes 2 cups. If making dressing, use an extra 1/2 to 1 cup of water.

GOLDEN GODDESS DRESSING

1/2 C organic cold-pressed flax oil
1/4 C fresh-squeezed lemon juice
1/4 C water
1-2 dates (soft varieties work better—honey,
    khadrawi, barhi, etc.)
1/2 C fresh cilantro
2 T Nama Shoyu
1 tsp sea salt
1-2 cloves garlic

Mix all ingredients in blender or food processor. Stores for only 2-3 days in refrigerator.

Variations - Use another fresh herb in place of cilantro.
    - Omit garlic for a garlic-free dressing.
    - Add a dash fresh-cracked black pepper.

BASIC TAHINI DRESSING

2/3 C raw sesame tahini
1 to 1 1/2 C water (depending on desired thickness)
1/4 C fresh lemon juice
1-2 cloves garlic
1 tsp sea salt
1 tsp Nama Shoyu
1 pitted date
1 very small pinch of cayenne pepper

Blend all ingredients in Vita-Mix or blender. Makes about 2 1/2 cups.

Variations - Try adding a bit of fresh parsley, scallions, or cumin.

TAHISO PASTE

3/4 C raw sesame tahini
3 T miso
2-3 T water

Mix all ingredients together with a wooden spoon until a consistent paste is made. This rich paste can be used as a dip for vegetables or a spread on crackers. It is a great fast protein food and it lasts for 3-4 weeks in the refrigerator.

BEAUTIFUL BEET DRESSING

1 beet, grated
3-4 cloves garlic
1/3 C olive oil
3 T raw apple cider vinegar
1/3 C water
2 tsp sea salt
1-2 pitted dates
1/2 tsp rosemary

Yes, beets are a hybridized food, and many raw-foodists try to avoid hybrids, but this is a very tasty dressing and one of my son's favorites (he'll try anything new with this dressing on it)—so I thought I'd include it. Just blend all of the ingredients in your blender or Vita-Mix and, voila! Makes 1 1/2 cups of brilliant fuchsia dressing—or try using a yellow beet and you'll have a vibrant golden dressing.

BASIC MISO DRESSING

1/4 C unpasteurized blonde miso
3 T apricot oil (or other mild oil of your choice)
1/2 C water
1 T Nama Shoyu
1 T raw apple cider vinegar

Mix all ingredients in food processor or blender. Makes 1 cup and stores well in refrigerator for a couple of weeks. This is my son's very favorite dressing!

Variations - try adding any of the following:
1 T chopped onion
1-2 cloves garlic
1 tsp fresh ginger
1/2 tsp orange zest or lemon zest
pinch of fresh-cracked black pepper
Or, try replacing the vinegar with lemon or orange juice.
If you would like to use a dark miso, add one pitted date.

SENSATIONAL CILANTRO DRESSING

1 bunch cilantro
3/4 C water
1/2 C macadamia nuts
1/4 C apricot oil (or other very mild oil of your choice)
2-3 cloves garlic
1 tsp fresh chopped ginger
1 1/2 tsp sea salt
juice of 1 lemon

Wash and de-stem the cilantro (this is the most time consuming part of the recipe). Mix all ingredients in your Vita-Mix or blender (you may have to add more water if using a regular blender). This is a very rich, delicious dressing that is reminiscent of Thai food.

Thank you, Marni for sharing your amazing cilantro pesto that inspired this dressing recipe. You are my favorite raw chef!

ASIAN DRESSING/MARINADE

3/4 C Nama Shoyu
1/4 C organic cold-pressed sesame oil
1/2 tsp fresh ginger
1 small clove garlic

Mix all ingredients in food processor or blender. Makes 1 cup. Stores well in refrigerator for a week or so.

This simple dressing makes an abundance of recipes comes to life, including Shredded Cabbage Salad (page 121), Stir-Not-Fried (page 133), and Asian Pasta (page 131).

Variations - add any of the following:
     red hot chili pepper
     cilantro
     fresh-ground black pepper
     fresh basil (esp. Thai basil)

Short-cut - Omega makes a Garlic/Chili flax oil that is very tasty. It's a great way to add flax oil to your diet. For a short cut to this marinade, mix 3/4 C Nama Shoyu and 1/4 C Garlic/Chili flax oil. It's a little on the fiery side, but oh so good!

BASIC VINAIGRETTE

1/4 C raw apple cider vinegar
1/2 C olive oil or other oil of your choice (alternate oils,
     they change the flavor a lot)
2 T water
1 tsp sea salt
1-2 cloves garlic, minced

Shake all ingredients in cruet, allow to sit for at least 15 minutes, then shake again before serving. Makes just less than 1 cup.

As the name states, this is a basic recipe and the variation possibilities are endless. Dried herbs do very well in this vinaigrette. Try adding one or more of the following:

1 tsp dried hot pepper, snipped in
1 tsp dried basil
1 tsp dried oregano
1 tsp dried thyme
1 tsp dried dill
1 tsp dried sage
1 tsp dried tarragon
1/2 tsp lemon, lime, orange or grapefruit zest
     (shavings of the rind)

BASIC CREAMY VINAIGRETTE

1/4 C raw apple cider vinegar
1/2 C olive oil or other oil of your choice
2 stalks celery
1 large or 2 small pitted dates
1 tsp sea salt
1-2 cloves garlic
1/2 C water

Blend all ingredients in food processor or blender, allow to sit for at least 15 minutes, then shake before serving. Makes 1 cup.

Another basic with lots of variation possibilities. Fresh herbs work wonderfully in this recipe. Try adding fresh marjoram, basil, cilantro, dill, parsley. My favorite for this recipe is 1/2 tsp rosemary (fresh or dried).

SALADS

POWERHOUSE KALE SALAD

1 large head kale (purple, red or Russian, dinosaur, etc.)
1/2 cucumber, chopped
1/2 red bell pepper, chopped
2 T olive oil
2 T raw apple cider vinegar
2 T Nama Shoyu
1-2 cloves garlic
1 T fresh basil or 1 tsp dried basil
1 T fresh oregano or 1 tsp dried oregano

Clean kale, remove hard stems and rip it into small bite-size pieces. Put all ingredients except cucumber and bell pepper into a bowl that is sealable. Seal the bowl and shake. Let the salad marinate at room temperature for 3 hours, and shake it every hour or so. Add the cucumber and bell pepper and let marinate for another 30 minutes. Serves 1-4, depending on whether it is a main or side dish. I always feel so energized after eating this salad!

ITALIAN CHOPPED SALAD

1 large head of lettuce, shredded
10 large basil leaves, chopped
10 kalamata olives, pitted and halved
1 small tomato, chopped
1 clove of garlic, minced
1 T apple cider vinegar
2 T olive oil
1 T Nama Shoyu

Shake all ingredients in a large bowl with lid. Serves 2-6, depending on whether it's a main course or side salad.

TOMATO CUCUMBER SALAD

4 tomatoes
2 cucumbers
1 C fresh basil
2 cloves garlic
sea salt to taste (optional)

This recipe can be made very quickly in a food processor, but can be made by hand too. Put garlic and basil in food processor and chop with s-blade. Take s-blade out (leaving chopped garlic and basil in the food processor). Put slicing blade on and alternately slice the tomatoes and cucumbers. Transfer to serving bowl. Mix gently. Sprinkle with sea salt and serve. Serves 2-6.

Variation - Instead of basil and garlic, use 1/4 C pitted and chopped kalamata olives. No sea salt for this variation.

CREAMY RED CABBAGE SALAD

1/2 head red cabbage, shredded
1 tomato chopped and drained
1-2 avocados, mashed
1/2 cucumber, chopped
1/2 red bell pepper, chopped
2 T chives, scallions, or red onion, chopped
2 cloves garlic
1 tsp cumin seeds
1 1/2 tsp ground cumin
2 T olive oil
1 tsp sea salt
juice of one lemon

Toss all ingredients, adding avocados last. Mix well.
Serves 2-4. This hearty salad holds up well, and leftovers can
be enjoyed for lunch the next day (if there are any leftovers!).

*Thank you, Marni & Korin for sharing your creamy cole slaw
that inspired this recipe.*

SHREDDED CABBAGE SALAD

1 head cabbage, shredded
4 stalks celery, thinly sliced
1/4 C sunflower seeds (or try sesame seeds or hemp seeds)
1/2 C Asian Dressing/Marinade (recipe page 115)

Shake all ingredients in a large bowl sealed with a lid. Remove lid and let sit for 5-10 minutes. Replace lid, shake again, and serve. Serves 4-10, depending on whether it is a main or side dish.

You can also toss just the cabbage and celery and keep in the refrigerator (will last for about 3-4 days) and add sunflower seeds and dressing to single servings shortly before you are going to eat them. This works great for brown bag lunches!

Variation - Serve over 1-2 cups of sprouted grains and increase the dressing by 1/4 to 1/2 cup.

PATES

WALNUT PATE
aka "tuna-salad"

3 C walnuts
2-3 cloves garlic
1 small onion (or half of a large one)
2-3 stalks celery
1/2 C fresh parsley
1 T fresh lemon juice
1-2 tsp sea salt

Soak walnuts for 30 minutes then drain. Put garlic, onion, celery and parsley into food processor and process with s-blade until the ingredients are finely chopped. Add walnuts, lemon juice and sea salt. Blend until smooth, "coaching" the mixing if necessary. Makes about 3 cups. You can add 1/2 C water to the paté and blend longer to create a dip.

Variation - Use fresh dill instead of parsley.

EASIEST MAC PATE

1 C macadamia nuts
1/2 chopped bell pepper – red, yellow, or orange

Process in food processor until a smooth consistency is achieved. Makes about 1 1/2 cups.

Variation - Use 1 cup chopped tomatillos instead of bell pepper.

HAZELNUT PATE

2 C hazelnuts
1 large tomato, cut into wedges
2 stalks celery, cut into large chunks
1 carrot, cut into large chunks
1 small red onion, cut into chunks
1/4 C fresh tarragon (or 2 T dried tarragon)
1 tsp ground cumin
1 tsp curry powder*
1/4 tsp ground cayenne
1-2 tsp sea salt
2 T fresh-squeezed lemon juice

Soak hazelnuts for 30 minutes then drain. Put tomato, celery, carrot, onion and tarragon into food processor and process with s-blade until the ingredients are finely chopped. Add hazelnuts, cumin, curry powder, cayenne, lemon juice and sea salt. Blend until smooth, "coaching" the mixing if necessary. Makes 3 cups.

* Traditional curry powder often contains toasted ingredients. If you cannot find a curry powder that has no toasted ingredients, add 1/2 tsp ground coriander and 1/2 tsp ground or fresh turmeric instead.

WALNUTFLOWER PATE

2 C walnuts
2 C cauliflower
1 clove garlic
1/4 tsp fresh ginger
2 T Nama Shoyu

Soak walnuts for 30 minutes then drain. Put cauliflower, garlic, and ginger into food processor and process with s-blade until the ingredients are finely chopped. Add walnuts and Nama Shoyu and blend until smooth, "coaching" the mixing if necessary. Makes 2 cups.

SUNFLOWER PATE

2 C sunflower seeds
2 small carrots, cut into chunks
1 clove garlic
1/4 tsp fresh ginger
2 T Nama Shoyu

Soak sunflower seeds for 30 minutes then drain. Put carrot, garlic, and ginger into food processor and process with s-blade until the ingredients are finely chopped. Add sunflower seeds and Nama Shoyu and blend until smooth. Add 2 T water, if necessary. Makes 2 cups.

KALAMATA TAPENADE

1 C walnuts, macadamias, or sunflower seeds (each impart a
    different flavor and each is delicious)
1 jar kalamata olives, drained and pitted
1 C sun-dried tomatoes
2 cloves garlic
1 T olive oil

Snip sun-dried tomatoes into smaller pieces (fours) with
your kitchen scissors. Soak in just enough water to cover and
set aside. Process nuts and garlic in food processor until they
become crumb-y. Add drained sun-dried tomatoes and pitted
kalamatas and process again. Scrape the sides of the food
processor down with a rubber spatula and process one last time,
adding the olive oil while the food processor is running. Makes
about 2 cups.

WALNUT PESTO

2 C walnuts
4 cloves garlic
2 C fresh basil, de-stemmed
1/2 C olive oil
pinch of sea salt (less than 1/4 tsp)

Process walnuts and garlic in food processor until they
become crumb-y. Add basil and process again. Scrape the
sides of the food processor down with a rubber spatula and process one last time, adding the olive oil and pinch of sea salt
while the food processor is running. Makes about 2 cups.

WHAT TO DO WITH PATES?

NORI ROLLS

1 C paté of your choice
1 cucumber, cut into long strips (exclude any portions
    containing seeds)
1 bunch scallions (optional)
1 1/2 C shredded vegetables (I usually use zucchini or
    yellow squash, but you can use any vegetable you like, or
    a combination)
1-2 ripe avocados, skins removed, sliced lengthwise
2 C shredded lettuce (or cabbage or other green)
2 C sunflower or other sprouts
6 raw nori sheets

Nori rolls have become a very popular raw-food dish and
they're not as hard to make as they may seem. You will need a
nori mat, which you can acquire at your food co-op or natural
food store, or an Asian market.

Place a raw nori sheet on the nori mat. About one inch
from the edge of the sheet closest to you, put a line of the paté.
Put a strip of cucumber on top of this and a scallion (optional).
Then layer avocado strips, shredded zucchini, shredded lettuce,
then sunflower sprouts. Dab end furthest from you with a bit
of water. Then use your mat to roll the nori sheet over the other
ingredients. Finish rolling by hand. Put nori roll to the side,
then when you are finished rolling all of your sheets, cut each
roll into 6 pieces. Makes 36 pieces.

NORI SNAPS

5 nori sheets
1/2 C paté of your choice

Using your kitchen scissors, cut each nori sheet into 16 squares (you can do a few layered sheets at a time). Put a tiny dollop of paté (about 1/2 teaspoon) into the center of a square. Dab the edges of the square with water (use your fingers to do this and get the nori sheet just barely moist). Put another square on top and press the edges. When you have made all of the squares, put them on trays in your dehydrator and dehydrate at 90 degrees for 4-5 hours. Makes 40 snaps. They are great little snacks to pack in lunches, serve with salads, and serve at parties. Store them in a brown paper bag and they can keep for up to a week. This recipe can be easily doubled or quadrupled.

DOLMAS

1 C paté of your choice (try the Hazelnut Paté)
1 C chopped tomatoes and cucumbers
10-15 young, soft chard leaves (older leaves are too
    brittle and will crack when you try to roll them)

This is a version of the stuffed grapeleaves I used to like so much. Trim the stems off the chard (save them for green juice or to snack on as-is). After cleaning, dry them very well, pressing them between clean towels to get all of the water off. Take a leaf, put a thick line of paté on the bottom or wider end, top with chopped tomatoes and cucumbers and roll. Makes 10-15 dolmas.

Variation - Use very large spinach leaves instead of chard.

STUFFED TOMATOES

20 large cherry tomatoes or 10 Roma tomatoes
1 C paté of your choice

If you are using large cherry tomatoes, cut the tops of and scoop out the seeds. Fill tomatoes with paté of your choice. If you are using Roma tomatoes, cut in half lengthwise, scoop out seeds, then fill with paté of your choice. Top with something decorative and complimentary: the top of a sunflower sprout, a cilantro leaf, a small radish wedge, etc. Serve as appetizers, snacks, or as a main dish over a bed of lettuce. Makes 20 stuffed tomatoes.

CUCUMBER POPPERS

1-2 cucumbers (peeled or not)
1 C paté of your choice

Cut cucumbers into slices about 1/4 inch thick. Top each cucumber slice with the paté of your choice, shaping the paté with a small spoon. Top with something decorative and complimentary: the top of a sunflower sprout, a cilantro leaf, a small radish wedge, etc. Serve as appetizers, snacks, or as a main dish over a bed of lettuce. Makes approximately 22 cucumber poppers.

Variation - Use zucchini or yellow summer squash instead of cucumbers.

A simple way to use paté - Use an ice-cream scooper to put scoops of paté on top of a big green salad.

RAWVIOLIS

2 medium turnips
1 C pate of your choice (the Walnut Pesto is the best for this)

"Rawviolis" has become another popular raw-food dish. Here is my recipe for them. Scrub the turnips clean. (It is not necessary to peel them.) Slice them in thin disks using a mandolin (see description in next section, The 21st Century Kitchen) or v-slicer. It may take a few times to get the hang of it and the right thickness. You want your disks to be thin and bendable. (If your turnip is too big for your mandolin, just slice one side. It is okay if your disks have a straight part.) Once you have sliced your turnips, place a small dab of pesto in each disk (about 1/2 T), fold in half and gently press. The pesto will make them "stick." Arrange them on a serving platter as you go. These are great for appetizers. To enjoy as a main course, serve over a bed of lettuce and pour a little Marinara Sauce (recipe page 131) on top.

STUFFED CELERY

4 stalks celery, cleaned and cut into 2 1/2" long pieces
1/2 C paté of your choice

Fill each piece of celery with paté, sprinkle with minced herbs, bell peppers, green onions, hemp seeds, or a combination, and serve. Makes approximately 20 stuffed celery pieces. This recipe is easy-as-can-be to make and always a favorite.

Variation - Use 4-5 young Belgian or French endive leaves (the non-curly type that looks like a fat cigar) instead of celery.

OTHER HEARTY FARE

"PASTA"

Raw pasta becomes miraculously easy with a little kitchen gadget called the Saladacco (see description in the next section, The 21st Century Kitchen). It makes long ribbons that resemble angel-hair pasta. Zucchini seems to be the biggest hit, but there are lots of other vegetables that will work, including turnips, rutabagas, large radishes, beets, carrots, etc. The amount of fruit or vegetables you need will depend on how many people you are serving and the size of the item you are making into the pasta (for example, some zucchini are very large and some are very small).

BETTER THAN ALFREDO SAUCE

2 C fresh cracked macadamia nuts
1/2 C pine nuts
2 T fresh squeezed lemon juice
3 cloves garlic
1 1/2 C water
1-2 T fresh de-stemmed thyme or 1 tsp dried thyme
1/4 small red hot chili pepper (optional)
1-2 tsp sea salt

Put macadamias, pine nuts, garlic, thyme, sea salt and water in Vita-Mix or blender. Use kitchen scissors to snip small pieces of the pepper into the blender or food processor. Blend until smooth, then add lemon juice and blend again. Makes 3 cups. Serve over pasta or a vegetable medley or add more water to make a creamy salad dressing.

MARINARA SAUCE

4 large tomatoes
3 T olive oil
1/4 C fresh cilantro
1/4 C fresh basil
2-3 cloves garlic
1 tsp dulse flakes
1 tsp ground cumin
2 tsp ground flax seed
4 pitted olives
1 pitted date
1-2 tsp sea salt

Slice tomatoes then put in a colander that is placed in a bowl. The bowl will catch the liquid from the tomatoes, which you can drink or add to a vegetable juice or save for another recipe. Let the tomatoes drain for 30 minutes to an hour. After the tomatoes have drained, put all ingredients into a food processor or blender and process just until smooth (you want your sauce to have body). It is best to wait an hour or so before serving so the flavors have a chance to meld. Makes 3 cups. Serve over pasta, use as a thick salad dressing or add tomato wedges and serve as a rich soup.

ASIAN PASTA

3 C zucchini pasta
1/2 C Asian Dressing (recipe page 115)
2 T hemp or sunflower seeds

Toss zucchini pasta and dressing. Sprinkle seeds on top and serve. Serves 2.

"MASHED POTATOES"

1 large head of cauliflower, cut into florets
2 C macadamia nuts

Put cauliflower and nuts through Champion using the blank plate or Green Star with tension knob off (you can also try using your food processor with the s-blade). Mix well with a wooden spoon. Makes 3-4 cups. The consistency is very similar to good old mashed potatoes. You can doctor this recipe up with garlic, lemon juice and minced chives or other herbs, or just leave it plain and top it with one of the following gravies.

GOURMET GRAVY

1 C Brazil nuts
1 avocado
2 T Nama Shoyu
2 T organic red wine
1 clove garlic
2 T chopped red onion
1-2 tsp sea salt
1 C water
pinch fresh-ground black pepper

Mix all ingredients in Vita-Mix or blender. Makes 2 1/2 cups. Serve over "Mashed Potatoes," a hearty vegetable pasta (turnip pasta for example), or a vegetable medley.

MINUTE GRAVY

Blend 1 T miso, 1 T nut or seed butter, and 1 cup water. OR Blend 1 T miso, 1/2 avocado and 1 cup water. Voila! Gravy in a minute!

MARINATED ASPARAGUS

1 bunch fresh asparagus
1 C Golden Goddess Dressing (recipe page 110)
1 head lettuce, shredded

Place asparagus in shallow container. Pour in dressing, making sure each stem is well-coated. Marinate at room temperature for 3 hours or in refrigerator for 6 hours or overnight. Take asparagus out of shallow container with tongs or fork and place on a bed of the shredded lettuce. Pour marinade over salad, amount depending on your taste.

STIR-NOT-FRIED

4 C broccoli, flowers and peeled stems
2 small carrots, shredded
1 C sunflower sprouts
5 small sunchokes, peeled and sliced (like water chestnuts)
1 C bok choy leaves
1/2 C Asian Dressing (recipe on page 115)

Shake all ingredients in a large bowl sealed with a lid. Remove lid and let sit for 30 minutes. Replace lid, shake again, and serve. Serves 4-10, depending on whether it is a main or side dish.

Variation - Serve over 1-2 cups of sprouted grains and increase the dressing by 1/4 to 1/2 cup.

ENCHILADAS or BURRITOS

Paté:
Easiest Mac Paté, recipe on page 122.

Filling:
4 cups of filling. Can be any of the following:
grated zucchini
grated yellow summer squash (crook-neck, sunburst, etc.)
fresh corn, cobbed
cilantro
olives
chopped tomatoes
chopped onions
mushrooms
avocado
chopped peppers

(Our family's favorite filling:
1 1/2 C grated zucchini
1 1/2 C fresh cobbed corn
1 1/2 C avocado--about 2 avocados
1/2 C destemmed cilantro)

    Put all filling ingredients in bowl. Mix and set aside.

Shells & toppings:
8 large lettuce leaves (for enchiladas)
or
8 large cabbage leaves (for burritos)

2 T chives

Sauce:
3 tomatoes
1 T mild oil
2 cloves garlic
1 tsp sea salt
1 pitted date
1/2 tsp ground cumin
1 1/2 tsp dried oregano
1/8 tsp ground cayenne pepper
1/16 tsp cinnamon

Chop the tomatoes then put them in a colander and let them drain for 30 minutes. Then mix all ingredients in your food processor or blender. Set aside.

If you're making enchiladas, put a line of paté in each leaf, add some of the filling mixture, then roll it and put on a serving plate. Cover with enchilada sauce and sprinkle with chopped chives. If you're making burritos, follow the same steps, except put the sauce and chives inside the shell before you roll it. Makes 8 enchiladas or burritos, serving 4-8.

Thank you, Holly, for a great dinner a couple of years ago and the idea of this recipe.

FALAFEL

1 1/2 C walnuts
1 1/2 C macadamia nuts
2 T chopped parsley
2 T chopped chives
2 T raw sesame tahini
1/4 C fresh lemon juice
1 clove garlic, minced
1 tsp ground cumin
1 tsp sea salt

Soak nuts for 15 minutes, then drain. Mix all ingredients with a wooden spoon in a large mixing bowl. Then put all ingredients through a Champion juicer with the blank plate, or a Green Power or Green Star with the tension nob removed. Add up to 1/2 cup water, if necessary. After processing, mix all ingredients thoroughly with clean hands.

With the falafel mixture, make a small ball (ping pong sized), then flatten the ball to make a patty. Put the patty on a mesh dehydrator tray. Continue until all the mixture is used up. Dehydrate for 8-10 hours at 95 degrees Fahrenheit. Makes 35-40 patties.

Serving suggestion - For shells, use large lettuce leaves (romaine and butter work best) and large purple cabbage leaves. Inside each shell, put 2-3 falafels, broken in half. Then put a couple of spoonfuls of Tomato Cucumber Salad (page 119, the variation with olives) and top with Basic Tahini Dressing (page 111).

FLAX CRACKERS

Tasty flax crackers are not only a great way to add flax to your diet, they can also take the place of chips and other crunchy snacks, filling a gap. Serve them with salads, raw soups, vegetable dips, or my favorite way to eat them is with plain avocado on top.

It may take a couple of tries to really get the hang of making flax crackers, but here is some information to help you get started.

Instead of soaking the flax seeds in water and then adding flavoring, I add the flavoring to the water, blending if necessary, before adding it to the flax seeds. This makes the flavors more evenly distributed and the whole process easier. A hint is that if you ever have extra vegetables or dip, you can blend them with your flax cracker liquid and go from there, fine-tuning the taste as necessary. Just be sure that if you have a lot of watery ingredients, you decrease the amount of water in your recipe.

When making flax crackers, you will spread the flax mixture on Teflex sheets, dehydrate for 2 hours or so, then transfer the flax cracker masses from the Teflex sheets to the mesh sheets. At this time, you can do a couple of things to make your flax crackers from more appealing to downright fancy. Usually you would just transfer the crackers and finish drying them, then you would break off pieces the way one does with Lavosh or Indian cracker breads. This is the easiest way. If however, you want a more uniform cracker, you can slice through the cracker mass with a pizza slicer or butter knife after you have transferred it to the mesh sheet, making squares.

This makes the crackers more appealing, especially to someone who may be turned off by the at-first funny look of flax crackers. If you want to get fancy (I have for parties), you can cut the flax cracker mass with cookie cutters in round or other shapes while it is still on the Teflex sheet. Transfer the cut shapes to the mesh sheets. Pile the "scraps" onto a mesh sheet (you can use these scraps for salads). Finish dehydrating.

I dehydrate at low temperatures to keep the food enzymes as intact as possible. A few years ago, I was wondering about how many enzymes really do make it through the dehydration process. I decided to do an experiment and I planted some of the flax crackers I had just made in some planting containers. About a month later I had flax plants everywhere! Their little blue blossoms were the prettiest in my container garden and a few months later, Stephen and I harvested the flax seeds.

One last tip is to chew, chew, chew your flax crackers! They can't be gobbled down the way traditional crackers can. You should also increase your fluid intake as flax seeds have so much soluble fiber.

The following recipes are for 4-5 trays of crackers and can be easily doubled to make 9 trays (which is what I usually make).

SAVORY FLAX CRACKERS

4 C flax seeds
2 C distilled water
1/2 of a leek
2 stalks celery
3/4 C walnuts
3-4 fresh sage leaves or 1 tsp dried sage
2 cloves garlic
1 T sea salt

Put flax seeds in large mixing bowl. Chop leek, celery, sage and garlic in blender or food processor. Add walnuts, chop again. Add this mixture, the water and the salt to the flax seeds and stir very well. Let sit for three hours, stirring every hour. After the flax seeds have soaked, spread the flax mixture onto Teflex sheets (or wax paper if you don't have Teflex sheets) with a rubber spatula. Put the Teflex sheets into the dehydrator and dehydrate for 2 hours at 95 degrees. After two hours, transfer the cracker spreads from the Teflex sheets to the mesh screens. (Do this by laying the mesh sheet on top of the cracker spreads, flipping the whole thing over and peeling off the Teflex sheet). Put the cracker spreads back into the dehydrator and dehydrate for 4-6 more hours at 95 degrees. When they are done, break them up into squares unless you have already shaped them. Store them in a brown paper bag.

PIZZA-FLAVORED FLAX CRACKERS

4 C flax seeds
1 C distilled water
1/2 zucchini
1-2 tomatoes
1/3 C pitted olives
2 tsp fresh or 1 tsp dried oregano
2 cloves garlic (optional)
1 T sea salt
1/2 tsp fennel seeds, ground

Put flax seeds in large mixing bowl. Chop zucchini, tomatoes, olives, oregano, fennel seeds and garlic in blender or food processor. Add this mixture, the water and the salt to the flax seeds and stir very well. Let sit for three hours, stirring every hour. After the flax seeds have soaked, spread the flax mixture onto Teflex sheets (or wax paper if you don't have Teflex sheets) with a rubber spatula. Put the Teflex sheets into the dehydrator and dehydrate for 2 hours at 95 degrees. After two hours, transfer the cracker spreads from the Teflex sheets to the mesh screens. (Do this by laying the mesh sheet on top of the cracker spreads, flipping the whole thing over and peeling off the Teflex sheet). Put the cracker spreads back into the dehydrator and dehydrate for 4-6 more hours at 95 degrees. When they are done, break them up into squares unless you have already shaped them. Store them in a brown paper bag.

SALSA FLAX CRACKERS

4 C flax seeds
1 C distilled water
1 C cilantro
1 red jalapeno pepper
2 tomatoes
1/2 small onion
2 T fresh-squeezed lemon juice
1 T sea salt
1/4 tsp ground cayenne pepper
1 clove garlic, optional

Put flax seeds in large mixing bowl. Chop cilantro, red pepper, tomato, and onion in blender or food processor. Add this mixture, the water and the salt to the flax seeds and stir very well. Let sit for three hours, stirring every hour. After the flax seeds have soaked, spread the flax mixture onto Teflex sheets (or wax paper if you don't have Teflex sheets) with a rubber spatula. Put the Teflex sheets into the dehydrator and dehydrate for 2 hours at 95 degrees. After two hours, transfer the cracker spreads from the Teflex sheets to the mesh screens. (Do this by laying the mesh sheet on top of the cracker spreads, flipping the whole thing over and peeling off the Teflex sheet). Put the cracker spreads back into the dehydrator and dehydrate for 4-6 more hours at 95 degrees. When they are done, break them up into squares unless you have already shaped them. Store them in a brown paper bag.

Short-cut - If you have access to raw, organic salsa, just blend 1 1/2 C salsa and 1/2 water, add to flax seeds, and go from there.

BEVERAGES & SWEETS

GOOD MORNING ALOE

1/3 giant aloe vera leaf, filleted (outer skin removed)
3 C fresh squeezed orange or other citrus juice

Blend both ingredients in Vita-mix or blender. Add ice if desired. Enjoy this creamy, satisfying drink as your first meal in the morning, or any time of day. Aloe has many healing properties and is especially helpful as an intestinal toner when ingested.

BASIC GREEN JUICE

5 handfuls kale or other green (spinach, chard,
    dandelion greens, collards, etc.)
1 cucumber
3 stalks celery

Put all foods through juicer and enjoy.

POWER GREEN JUICE

3 handfuls one kind of green
3 handfuls another kind of green
1 cucumber
3 stalks celery
2 handfuls parsley
1-2 T Nature's First Food superfood

Put greens, cucumber, celery and parsley through juicer. Stir in Nature's First Food.

GREAT V-8 ALIKE

5 handfuls red chard
3 handfuls spinach
1 cucumber
2 stalks celery
2 tomatoes
1 red pepper (bell, jalapeno, etc.)
1 clove garlic
2 T dulse

Put all ingredients except dulse through juicer. Put juice and dulse into Vita-Mix or blender. Let sit for five minutes (to soften dulse) then blend. Voile! Tastes so much like commercial V-8!

BASIC SMOOTHIE

1 C fresh fruit juice
1 frozen banana
1 C fresh or frozen fruit

Mix all ingredients in Vita-Mix or blender and enjoy!

BEST POWER SMOOTHIE

1 C fresh orange or other fruit juice
1 frozen banana
1 C fresh or frozen berries
3 T goji berries
1 T NFL tocotrienols
1 T Truly Natural Vitamin C powder

Mix all ingredients in Vita-Mix or blender and enjoy!

ABC SMOOTHIE

2 C fresh apple juice
2 frozen bananas
meat from 2 young coconuts

Mix all ingredients in Vita -Mix or blender and enjoy!

LASSI SMOOTHIE

2 C fresh orange juice
3 C fresh or frozen mangoes
2 T macadamia nuts

Mix all ingredients in Vita-Mix or blender and enjoy!

VENUS SMOOTHIE

1 C fresh orange juice
1 frozen banana
3 T flax seeds
1 T bee pollen
1 T Truly Natural Vitamin C
3 ice cubes

This smoothie is my favorite pregnancy power smoothie (nursing too) as it has staying power and is high in the vitamins, minerals, protein and essential fatty acids that are all so important during pregnancy and breastfeeding. Of course, it will be beneficial to non-pregnant and non-lactating persons too!

Mix all ingredients except the banana and ice cubes in your Vita-Mix. Once the flax seeds are broken up and mixed well, add the banana and ice cubes. Enjoy!

APPLE PIE SMOOTHIE

2 C fresh apple juice
1 C pecans (soaked for 30 minutes)
1 fresh or frozen banana (optional)
3 pitted dates
1/8 tsp cinnamon

Mix all ingredients in Vita-Mix or blender and enjoy!

ORANGE JULIA

2 C fresh squeezed orange juice
3 T almond butter
3 large pitted dates
1 C water

Blend all ingredients in Vita-Mix or blender until smooth and frothy. If you like your drinks cold, you can add 2 ice cubes before blending. Serves 1-2.

Short-cut - Blend equal parts fresh orange juice and nut milk and a couple of ice cubes.

PECAN MILK

3/4 C pecans
3 C water
4 pitted dates (optional)

Mix all ingredients in blender or Vita-Mix. Makes about 4 cups.

MAC MILK

1 C macadamia nuts
3 C water
1-5 large dates, pitted (optional)

Mix all ingredients in food processor or blender. If you like you nut milk thicker, add less water. Makes 4 cups.

Note - Many people strain their nut milks but I have never found it necessary.

MAC PUDDING

3/4 C macadamia nuts (or try cashews)
1 C blueberries or strawberries, fresh or frozen
8 large dates, pitted
1 1/4 C water

Blend dates and water until smooth. Add berries and blend again. Add macadamia nuts slowly, blending as you go, coaching the mixing if necessary. Eat as-is or dip cut-up fruit in (apples are especially tasty dipped in this pudding).

COCONUT CUSTARD

Coconut meat from 4-5 young coconuts
1 vanilla bean
10-20 dates (depending on the size and sweetness
    of the dates you are using)
1 1/2 C water

Pit dates and soak them in the water for 30 minutes or so (you can have them soaking while you remove the meat from the coconuts). Put water and dates into Vita-Mix or blender. Snip in vanilla bean with kitchen scissors. Blend until smooth. Start adding coconut meat and blend. You coax your blender through this recipe by stirring in between blending and scraping the sides with a spatula. You may also have to add a little more water. Best when served chilled. Makes 3 1/2 cups, which can serve 2-8, depending on whether it's dessert or a meal! You can replace the water in this recipe with the water from the coconut; it gives the custard a whole different taste.

RECIPES FROM RAW POWER! 1st EDITION

CAPTAIN'S POWERHOUSE

1 young coconut
1 large avocado
2 handfuls wild or organic greens

Drain coconut water into Vita-Mix or blender. Crack coconut in half, scoop out the soft meat and add to Vita-Mix. Scoop avocado with spoon and add to Vita-Mix. Add two handfuls of greens. Blend until smooth. (Drink 30 minutes after work-out for best results.)

GO-THROUGH-A-BRICK-WALL JUICE

6 ounces sprouted wheatberries
6 handfuls of wild or organic dandelion greens
1 ounce ginger root

Put 3-day sprouted wheatberries through juicer. (For information on how to sprout wheat, read "The Wheatgrass Book" by Ann Wigmore.) Put ginger through juicer. Put greens through juicer. Pour juice into large glass. This drink is electrical—quite a jolt!

THE PROTEIN MYTH

5 ounces wheatgrass juice
the milk (or water) from 1 young coconut

Put wheatgrass through Miracle Wheatgrass Juicer until you have 5 ounces of juice. Pour into large glass. Add water from young coconut and drink!

FIRE WATER

1 orange or red habanero pepper
1 medium orange
4 cups distilled water

Put habanero pepper in juicer. Peel orange and discard orange peel. Put orange fruit through juicer. Pour 4 cups of distilled water into juicer to flush out remaining nutrients. Pour Fire Water into pitcher and serve. It is best to drink this 30 minutes before a meal.

POST-WORK-OUT DRINK

3 stalks celery
2 medium apples

Put foods through juicer. Drink after your work-out. Excellent sodium/potassium balance.

DATENUT SHAKE

1 cup soaked almonds (or other nut of your choice)
4-6 dates
distilled water

Remove and discard date pits. Blend soaked almonds and date fruits with distilled water to desired consistency.

CW TRAIL MIX

1/2 C macadamias
1/2 C pistachios
1/2 C raisins (with seeds)
1/2 C dried apricots
1/2 C seaweed (laver or dulse)

Mix all together in a bag (powerful combo!).

AVO SOUP

2 large avocados
1 medium cucumber
1 medium tomato
1/2 C loose corn
1 C chopped zucchini
1/4 C chopped green onion
1 T fresh cilantro
distilled water

Discard avocado pits and skins. Put 1-1/2 avocado, cucumber, tomato, and cilantro into blender. Blend, adding distilled water for desired consistency. Pour into a bowl. Chop remaining 1/2 avocado into small cubes and stir into soup, along with the zucchini, corn, and onions.

FATS AVOCADO SALAD

3-4 handfuls wild or organic greens
2 large avocados
30-40 Raw Power! Olives
1 T extra-virgin cold-pressed olive oil
1 medium orange

Discard pits of olives, pits and skins of avocados, and orange peel. Make a bed of wild or organic greens and/or herbs, add avocado, olives, olive oil, and add juice of the orange to taste. Greens and fats are your body-builders. Powerful salad!

APPLENUT SALAD

1 head red leaf lettuce
1 cup sunflower sprouts
1 diced apple
1/2 cup chopped walnuts
1 cup grapes

Make a bed of lettuce and sprouts. Put apple, walnuts, and grapes on top of bed.

BACHELOR BURRITOS

4 large avocados
1 medium red onion, diced
3 red jalapeno peppers, seeded and diced
1 head red cabbage
2 yellow limes

Mix ingredients avocados (skins and pits removed), onion and jalapeno peppers. This is your burrito filler. Spoon out filler into unbroken red cabbage leaves, squeeze lime juice onto filler, and wrap each leaf around filler to create "raw burritos."

ANTS IN A CANOE

2 large apples
2 cups soaked almonds
2 ounces raisins (with seeds)

Soak almonds in distilled water for 12 hours. Put soaked almonds through a Champion or Green Power Juicer, using the blank plate. This will make almond butter. Cut apples into quarters. Remove and discard seeds. Spread almond butter on apples then cover with raisins. Great snack. (Kelly Alexander taught me this one.)

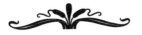

The 21st Century Kitchen
by Jolie

Below is a list of items that can help you establish your raw, living-foods kitchen. Items in **bold** are available from Nature's First Law (www.rawfood.com).

<u>Bag tree</u> — This is a little wooden tree that makes recycling plastic bags easy. Just turn your produce and ziplock bags inside out, quickly rinse off if necessary, and put them on the bag tree to dry out.

<u>Baskets</u> — You'll want lots of baskets for your produce. Try to procure shallow square baskets in varying sizes, so your produce doesn't have to sit on top of each other. If you have a pest or space problem, hanging baskets are a great solution. Hanging basket sets are usually three-tiered and are hung from the ceiling with a plant-hanging hook.

<u>Blender - heavy duty</u> — I recommend the **Vita-Mix** blender. Most blenders have 1/16 horsepower motors while the Vita-Mix has a 2.014 horsepower motor that the makers claim can grind a 2x4 wooden block into sawdust! Once you have tried a Vita-Mix, you won't want to go back to using a regular blender. It makes the best smoothies on earth and can make smooth, tasty drinks of raw fruits and veggies even without removing the seeds or skin. It is perfect for "liquid salads" or raw soups. This is my most-used kitchen appliance.

<u>Bowls</u> — A good set of bowls is essential for food preparation and serving. Wooden, glass, ceramic or terra cotta bowls are

all preferable to plastic or metal. Make sure you have good-sized bowls for your salads. Traditional "salad bowls" are small and intended for side salads, not meal salads. If you get a nice set or two of bowls that nestle, it will save space in your kitchen.

Colanders and strainers of varying sizes. (Ceramic or terra cotta best, stainless steel next best.)

Cutting boards — Wooden are preferable to plastic. Have a separate one for onions, garlic and other savory items. Care for your cutting boards and other wooden items by oiling them properly and often. I oil mine with olive oil – which makes for a good hand-treatment too!

Dehydrator — It is best to sun-dry when you can, but there are few locations where this is practical, and even in these locations, there are only a few months hot and dry enough for sun-drying. A dehydrator is great for drying produce for later consumption (perfect for when you have excess produce that will otherwise go bad), making flax crackers (a great replacement for chips!), and lots of other fun recipes. Nature's First Law offers the **Excalibur 5-tray and 9-tray dehydrators**. The 5-tray is practical if you are preparing for only 1 or 2 people, otherwise, the 9-tray is recommended. The Excalibur is the best dehydrator I've tried. It's easy to clean, has a good fan system, and has temperature control from 85 to 145 F (I don't dehydrate higher than 95 F). The shelves and mesh screens that come with the Excalibur can also be used for sun-drying. **Teflex sheets** keep wet or gooey food from slipping through small holes in the dehydrator trays. These are key for dehydrating crackers, desserts, etc.

Flax Seed Grinder — The grinder Nature's First Law carries is specially designed to grind up flax seeds. It makes adding flax to your diet simple and easy. The milling/grinding surface is ceramic and has 3 adjustable settings. You can also use the flax seed grinder for other seeds like sesame, fennel, cardamom, cumin, etc.

Food Processor — I have preferred Cuisinart food processors. Models that can slice, dice, grate as well as chop, pulse and homogenize are the best.

Funnels of varying sizes. These are used to transfer dressings and other liquids to their serving and storing containers.

Garlic press — This little device makes garlic mincing quick and easy.

Glassware — Big rectangular dishes, pie dishes, bowls, etc. Glassware is easy to clean and superior to plastic.

Glass Bottles & Jars — Recycled glass bottles with plastic lids are great for food storage (the glass bottle doesn't off-gas or leach the way plastic does and the plastic lid—which doesn't actually touch your food—doesn't rust the way metal lids do). I know, I know, you don't use processed commercial foods anymore, but surely you have a friend or relative who still does. Ask them to save their glass bottles with plastic lids for you—especially ones for salad dressing. Canning or Mason jars are great for storing and transporting food, too. They can also be used for soaking and sprouting nuts and seeds. Take care to wash the two-part lids well and dry them quickly so they don't rust. If you ever come across a plastic lid that fits these bottles, hang onto it!

Hand food processor — One with multiple grating and slicing options is the best. Mine is the "grinder" type with five different grinding cones.

Juicers, Juicers, Juicers!

We have lots of juicers in our house and we really do use them all. They each have different benefits in use. Hopefully the descriptions below will help you decide which juicer(s) will fit your needs.

Champion Juicer (Commercial Model) — The Champion Juicer is a "mastication" juicer. Makes raw "ice cream," patés, dips, etc. (In fact, most people I know who have Champions use them more as food-processors than juicers.) The Champion chews and presses the fibers and breaks up the cells of fruits and vegetables. This gives you more fiber, enzymes, vitamins, and trace minerals. The Champion's body is lined with a special stainless steel, which is almost wear-free and will not pick up food odors. Versatile, easy to use, relatively easy to clean.

Citrus juicer — I have liked the Braun models the best. Having a citrus juicer makes juicing citrus a breeze and can be used by older children (after they have been shown how to use it safely). A hand citrus juicer is also recommended for making small amounts of juices for recipes and for travel or the office.

Green Power Juicer — This is one of the best juicers on the market today. The Green Power has a twin-gear, low-RPM motor that produces less heat, which minimizes loss of nutrition. The slow-moving triturating twin gears crush fruits and vegetables, rather than cutting them. This machine expels a drier pulp, an indication that more juice and more nutrients are being extracted. Green juice made with this juicer is more mineral-rich than other green juices, a fact made obvious by the non-bitter taste. The **Green Star Juicer** has the same functions as the Green Power, only is more compact (and has a better warranty).

Juiceman II — This is the most convenient and easy-to-use juicer available. It offers a powerful motor with built-in speed control for optimum extraction efficiency. Great for making lots of juice (for families or parties) in the least amount of time. It is especially good for making apple, pear and melon juices. The **Juiceman Jr.** is great "starter" juicer. It is also good for travelling or taking to the office as it is so small, light, and easy to clean.

Miracle Wheatgrass Juicer (electric) — Wheatgrass is a quick, easy, inexpensive way to add chlorophyll and other minerals and vitamins to your diet. I think it's the best replacement for that cup of coffee in the morning and it keeps you going much longer! There are also countless applications for wheatgrass that go far beyond drinking it. (For more information, read Ann Wigmore's **The Wheatgrass Book**.) In addition to juicing wheatgrass, you can also use this juicer for berries, leafy greens, and grapes. The manual **Miracle Wheatgrass Juicer** is the manual version of the electric juicer made of tin-plated cast iron. It can be attached to any counter-type surface.

Knives — A good knife set is essential and can make food preparation quick and easy. Dull, flimsy knives or using the wrong knife for the job can make food prep slow, difficult, and dangerous. Take care of your knives by not soaking them in water, not putting them in the dishwasher, and sharpening your metal knives every other month or so. **Ceramic Knives** are neat because they decrease oxidation of the food being cut. I was initially skeptical about ceramic knives so I performed a little test, cutting one apple with my regular metal knife and cutting another apple with a ceramic knife. The apple cut with the metal knife turned brown (oxidized) within minutes. The apple cut with the ceramic knife did not turn color for hours, and even then it was only slightly changed. I think it is wise to have ceramic knives for cutting produce. The only drawback to the ceramic knife is that it is a little on the fragile side and it doesn't work as well on thick root vegetables (turnips, sunchokes, etc.).

Mandoline or V-slicer — Nature's First Law carries the **Mandoline Plus**, a practical kitchen tool for slicing and shredding vegetables. It comes with three stainless steel shredding blades, a stationary cutting blade, an adjustable platform, a finger guard, and a clear plastic catch tray with grater. There are many different types of mandolines on the market, but this one is the best because it is the safest and the container on the bottom catches the sliced or shredded food, eliminating the mess most mandolines make. It slices very, very thin! (Hint - you can slice cucumbers or zucchini on their sides, then wrap these long, thin rectangular slices around pate and sprouts or shredded veggies for an incredibly fresh wrap snack!)

Mortar and pestle — Use for grinding seeds or other items into powder.

Nutcracker — Nature's First Law carries the **Krakanut**, "The World's Finest Nutcracker." It really is too. It cracks the hardest nuts (macadamias, black walnuts, hickorynuts, butternuts, etc.) perfectly every time with no mess, yet it can also be used on soft nuts like pecans. Whenever possible, I crack the nuts I use in my recipes for increased flavor and nutrition. The Krakanut makes it so much easier. (I used to use a brick on the patio to crack our macadamias!) It is also fun for older kids to crack their own nuts (after they have been shown how to use the nutcracker safely), and there have been lots of parties where I have just put out the Krakanut and a bowl of nuts to keep everyone happily occupied while I finished up in the kitchen.

Rubber spatulas — these are used to scrape out dressings, patés, smoothies, and sauces from the food processor bowl and Vita-Mix. Also key for spreading flax crackers on Teflex sheets.

Salad spinner — For anyone frequently making and eating salad, a salad spinner is very handy. There are lots of different models, from a grinder handle type to a lawnmower pull mechanism type (I always get a laugh when I use my friend's lawnmower type salad spinner!). I prefer the kind where you just push down on a big knob. I have the OXO Good Grips model.

Scissors — You should have a pair of scissors designated as "Kitchen Only" scissors (you can even write that on the handle to remind others). Kitchen scissors can be used for snipping fresh vanilla bean, fresh or dried chiles and peppers (this saves your fingers from those little burns), fresh or dried herbs, and seaweed right into your recipes.

Spiralizer — Nature's First Law carries the **Saladacco Spiralizer**. This gadget makes the most incredible raw angelhair pasta by spiralizing zucchini and other vegetables into thin, long strings. Add a little raw pesto or other sauce and you are ready for a meal! You can also make long ribbons for decorating your dishes.

Sprouter — If you enjoy sprouts, but are intimidated by sprouting, try the **EasyGreen Front Loader**. It has been called "the best automatic home sprouter in the world" and is the newest design for starting virtually every sproutable seed. Complete with a mist generator, timer, five cartridges, an owner's manual, collection pan, and drain tube. The EasyGreen Front Loader is ready to use. Just add water and seeds. This model is suitable for stacking.

Water Distiller — Distilled water is important for drinking and using in recipes when you can't get other highly purified water. You can revitalize your distilled water by placing it in a big glass container with a quartz crystal in the bottom, by putting a blade or two of wheatgrass in your container of water, or by adding a bit of fresh-squeezed lemon juice. Nature's First Law offers the **EcoWater Distiller**. This model is a one-gallon home distiller and is completely portable. (Distillers have come a long way—I remember the distiller my grandpa had when I was growing up, it was as big as a kitchen stove!) It is very easy to use. Just fill with one gallon of water and plug into a 120 volt outlet. Produces one gallon of distilled water in four hours. Automatically shuts off when the cycle is complete.

Wooden spoons — have an assortment of wooden spoons for stirring, mixing, and salad tossing. Care for them in the same manner as your cutting boards and wooden bowls by cleaning them well, not soaking them in water, and oiling them regularly. (By doing this, I've had the same set of wooden spoons for over ten years!)

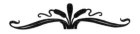

Work-Outs

MEN'S STANDARD WORK-OUT

Monday / Wednesday / Friday

WARM-UP

<u>Neck Rolls</u>: 5 rolls to each side
<u>Side Bends</u>: 10 reps to each side
<u>Lunges/Achilles Stretches</u>: 5 combinations
<u>Windmills</u>: 20 reps to each side

CHEST

<u>Barbell Bench Press</u>: 5 sets + warm-up set
  1 set of 15 rep warm-up
  sets of 10,8,6,4,4 reps - stripping last two sets
<u>Incline Barbell Bench Press</u>: 5 sets
  sets of 10,8,6,4,4 reps - stripping last two sets
<u>Dumbbell Flys</u>: 5 sets
  sets of 10,8,8,8,6 reps
<u>Parallel Dips</u>: 5 sets
  sets of 15,10,8,8,8 reps
<u>Dumbbell Pullovers</u>: 3 sets
  sets of 15,15,15 reps

BACK

<u>Wide-Grip Chin-Ups</u>: 5 sets
  10 reps first 3 sets, go until failure last 2 sets

Close-Grip Chin-Ups: 5 sets
  10 reps each set
T-Bar Rows: 5 sets
  sets of 15,12,10,8,6 reps
Bent-Over Barbell Rows: 5 sets
  10 reps each set

THIGHS

Squats: 5 sets + warm-up set
  1 set of 20 rep warm-up
  sets of 10,8,6,4,4 reps
Front Squats: 4 sets
  sets of 10,8,8,6 reps
Hack Squats: 4 sets
  10 reps each set
Lying Leg Curls: 5 sets
  sets of 20,10,8,6,6 reps
Standing Leg Curls: 5 sets
  10 reps each set
Straight-Leg Deadlifts: 3 sets
  10 reps each set

CALVES

Donkey Calf Raises: 5 sets
  10 reps each set
Standing Calf Raises: 5 sets
  sets of 15,10,8,8,8 reps

ABDOMINALS

Bent-Knee Hanging Leg Raises: 100 reps
Bent-Over Twists: 100 reps each side
Crunches: 50 reps

CARDIOVASCULAR

<u>Walk, Run, Bike, Swim, or Hike</u>: 30-60 minutes

Tuesday / Thursday / Saturday

WARM-UP

<u>Neck Rolls</u>: 5 rolls to each side
<u>Side Bends</u>: 10 reps to each side
<u>Lunges/Achilles Stretches</u>: 5 combinations
<u>Windmills</u>: 20 reps to each side

SHOULDERS

<u>Behind-Neck Barbell Presses</u>: 4 sets + warm-up
  1 set of 15 rep warm-up
  sets of 10,8,8,6 reps
<u>Dumbbell Lateral Raises</u>: 5 sets
  8 reps each set
<u>Bent-Over Lateral Raises</u>: 5 sets
  8 reps each set
<u>Dumbbell Shrugs</u>: 3 sets
  10 reps each set

UPPER ARMS

<u>Standing Barbell Curls</u>: 5 sets
  sets of 15,10,8,6,4 reps
<u>Incline Dumbbell Curls</u>: 5 sets
  8 reps each set
<u>Concentration Curls</u>: 3 sets
  8 reps each set

Lying French Presses: 5 sets
  sets of 15,10,8,6,4 reps
Triceps Cable Pushdowns: 5 sets
  8 reps each set
One-Arm Triceps Extensions: 5 sets
  10 reps each set

FOREARMS

Barbell Wrist Curls: 5 sets
  10 reps each set
Reverse Wrist Curls: 3 sets
  10 reps each set

CALVES

Seated Calf Raises: 5 sets
  10 reps each set

ABDOMINALS

Bent-Knee Sit-Ups: 100 reps
Incline Board Leg Raises: 100 reps

CARDIOVASCULAR

Walk, Run, Bike, Swim, or Hike: 30-60 minutes

MEN'S ADVANCED WORK-OUT

Monday / Wednesday / Friday

WARM-UP

<u>Neck Rolls</u>: 5 rolls to each side
<u>Side Bends</u>: 10 reps to each side
<u>Lunges/Achilles Stretches</u>: 5 combinations
<u>Windmills</u>: 20 reps to each side

ABDOMINALS

<u>Roman Chair Sit-Ups</u>: 5 minutes

CHEST & BACK

Superset:
<u>Barbell Bench Press</u>: 5 sets + warm-up set
  1 set of 15 rep warm-up
  sets of 10,8,6,4,4 reps
<u>Wide-Grip Chin-Ups</u>: 5 sets
  10 reps each set

Superset:
<u>Dumbbell Incline Presses</u>: 5 sets
  sets of 10,8,8,8,6 reps
<u>Close-Grip Chin-Ups</u>: 5 sets
  10 reps each set
<u>Dumbbell Flys</u>: 5 sets
  sets of 10,8,8,8,6 reps
<u>Parallel Dips</u>: 5 sets
  sets of 15,10,8,8,8 reps

T-Bar Rows: 5 sets
  sets of 15,10,8,8,8 reps
Bent-Over Barbell Rows: 5 sets
  10 reps each set

Superset:
Seated Cable Rows: 5 sets
  10 reps each set
Dumbbell Pullovers: 5 sets
  15 reps each set

THIGHS

Squats: 6 sets
  sets of 15,10,8,8,6,4 reps
Front Squats: 4 sets
  sets of 10,8,8,6 reps

Superset:
Hack Squats: 5 sets + warm up set
  1 set of 15 rep warm-up
  sets of 10,8,8,8,8 reps
Lying Leg Curls: 5 sets + warm-up set
  1 set of 15 rep warm-up
  sets of 10,8,8,8,8 reps

Superset:
Standing Leg Curls: 5 sets
  10 reps each set
Straight-Leg Deadlifts: 5 sets
  10 reps each set

CALVES

Donkey Calf Raises: 5 sets
  10 reps each set
Standing Calf Raises: 5 sets
  10 reps each set
Seated Calf Raises: 5 sets
  10 reps each set

ABDOMINALS

Bent-Knee Hanging Leg Raises: 150 reps
Crunches: 150 reps
Bent-Over Twists: 100 reps each side

CARDIOVASCULAR

Walk, Run, Bike, Swim, or Hike: 30-60 minutes

Tuesday / Thursday / Saturday

WARM-UP

Neck Rolls: 5 rolls to each side
Side Bends: 10 reps to each side
Lunges/Achilles Stretches: 5 combinations
Windmills: 20 reps to each side

ABDOMINALS

Roman Chair Sit-Ups: 5 minutes

SHOULDERS

Superset:
<u>Behind-Neck Barbell Presses</u>: 5 sets + warm-up set
  1 set of 15 rep warm-up
  sets of 10,8,8,8,6 reps
<u>Dumbbell Lateral Raises</u>: 5 sets
  8 reps each set

Superset:
<u>Machine Front Press</u>: 5 sets
  8 reps each set
<u>Bent-Over Lateral Raises</u>: 5 sets
  8 reps each set

Superset:
<u>Upright Rows</u>: 5 sets
  10 reps each set
<u>One-Arm Seated Cable Laterals</u>: 5 sets
  10 reps each set, each arm

UPPER ARMS

Superset:
<u>Standing Barbell Curls</u>: 5 sets
  sets of 15,10,8,6,4 reps
<u>Lying French Presses</u>: 5 sets
  sets of 15,10,8,6,4 reps

Superset:
<u>Alternate Dumbbell Curls</u>: 5 sets
  8 reps each set
<u>Triceps Cable Pushdowns</u>: 5 sets
  8 reps each set

Superset:
Concentration Curls: 5 sets
  8 reps each set
One-Arm Triceps Extensions: 5 sets
  12 reps each set
Reverse Push-Ups: 5 sets
  15 reps each set

FOREARMS

Superset:
Barbell Wrist Curls: 5 sets
  10 reps each set
Reverse Wrist Curls: 5 sets
  10 reps each set
One-Arm Wrist Curls: 5 sets
  10 reps each set

CALVES

Standing Calf Raises: 5 sets
  sets of 15,10,8,8,8 reps
Calf Raises On Leg Press Machine: 5 sets
  10 reps each set

ABDOMINALS

Bent-Knee Sit-Ups: 150 reps
Incline Board Leg Raises: 150 reps
Side Leg Raises: 100 reps each side
Hyperextensions: 3 set
  10 reps each set

CARDIOVASCULAR

<u>Walk, Run, Bike, Swim, or Hike</u>: 30-60 minutes

WOMEN'S STANDARD WORK-OUT

Monday / Wednesday / Friday

WARM-UP

Neck Rolls: 5 rolls to each side
Side Bends: 10 reps to each side
Lunges/Achilles Stretches: 5 combinations
Windmills: 20 reps to each side

CHEST

Barbell Bench Press: 4 sets + warm-up set
  1 set of 15 rep warm-up
  sets of 12,10,8,6 reps
Incline Barbell Bench Press: 4 sets
  sets of 12,10,8,8 reps
Dumbbell Flys: 4 sets
  sets of 10,8,8,8 reps
Dumbbell Pullovers: 3 sets
  sets of 12,12,12 reps

BACK

Lat Machine Pulldowns: 4 sets
  sets of 15,12,10,8 reps
Lat Machine Pulldowns - Close-Grip: 4 sets
  sets of 15,12,10,8 reps
Bent-Over Barbell Rows: 3 sets
  10 reps each set

THIGHS

<u>Squats</u>: 3 sets + warm-up set
  1 set of 20 rep warm-up
  sets of 12,10,8 reps
<u>Hack Squats</u>: 4 sets
  10 reps each set
<u>Lying Leg Curls</u>: 5 sets
  sets of 20,10,8,6,6 reps
<u>Standing Leg Curls</u>: 5 sets
  10 reps each set

CALVES

<u>Standing Calf Raises</u>: 5 sets
  sets of 15,10,8,8,8 reps

ABDOMINALS

<u>Bent-Knee Hanging Leg Raises</u>: 50 reps
<u>Bent-Over Twists</u>: 100 reps each side
<u>Crunches</u>: 100 reps

CARDIOVASCULAR

<u>Walk, Run, Bike, Swim, or Hike</u>: 30-60 minutes

Tuesday / Thursday / Saturday

WARM-UP

<u>Neck Rolls</u>: 5 rolls to each side
<u>Side Bends</u>: 10 reps to each side
<u>Lunges/Achilles Stretches</u>: 5 combinations
<u>Windmills</u>: 20 reps to each side

SHOULDERS

<u>Behind-Neck Barbell Presses</u>: 4 sets + warm-up
  1 set of 15 rep warm-up
  sets of 12,10,8,8 reps
<u>Dumbbell Lateral Raises</u>: 4 sets
  8 reps each set
<u>Bent-Over Lateral Raises</u>: 4 sets
  8 reps each set
<u>Dumbbell Shrugs</u>: 3 sets
  10 reps each set

UPPER ARMS

<u>Standing Barbell Curls</u>: 4 sets
  sets of 12,10,8,6 reps
<u>Incline Dumbbell Curls</u>: 4 sets
  8 reps each set
<u>Concentration Curls</u>: 3 sets
  8 reps each set
<u>Lying French Presses</u>: 4 sets
  sets of 12,10,8,6 reps
<u>Triceps Cable Pushdowns</u>: 4 sets
  8 reps each set
<u>One-Arm Triceps Extensions</u>: 3 sets
  10 reps each set

FOREARMS

<u>Barbell Wrist Curls</u>: 4 sets
  10 reps each set
<u>Reverse Wrist Curls</u>: 3 sets
  10 reps each set

CALVES

Seated Calf Raises: 4 sets
  10 reps each set

ABDOMINALS

Bent-Knee Sit-Ups: 100 reps
Incline Board Leg Raises: 50 reps

CARDIOVASCULAR

Walk, Run, Bike, Swim, or Hike: 30-60 minutes

WOMEN'S ADVANCED WORK-OUT

Monday / Wednesday / Friday

WARM-UP

Neck Rolls: 5 rolls to each side
Side Bends: 10 reps to each side
Lunges/Achilles Stretches: 5 combinations
Windmills: 20 reps to each side

ABDOMINALS

Roman Chair Sit-Ups: 5 minutes

CHEST & BACK

Superset:
Barbell Bench Press: 5 sets + warm-up set
  1 set of 15 rep warm-up
  sets of 12,10,8,6,4 reps
Lat Machine Pulldowns: 5 sets
  sets of 12,10,8,8,6 reps

Superset:
Dumbbell Incline Presses: 5 sets
  sets of 12,10,8,8,6 reps
Lat Machine Pulldowns - Close Grip: 5 sets
  sets of 12,10,8,8,6 reps
Dumbbell Flys: 5 sets
  sets of 10,8,8,8,6 reps
Parallel Dips: 5 sets
  sets of 15,10,8,8,8 reps

Bent-Over Barbell Rows: 5 sets
  10 reps each set

Superset:
Seated Cable Rows: 5 sets
  10 reps each set
Dumbbell Pullovers: 5 sets
  15 reps each set

THIGHS

Squats: 6 sets
  sets of 15,10,8,8,6,6 reps
Front Squats: 4 sets
  sets of 10,8,8,6 reps

Superset:
Hack Squats: 5 sets + warm up set
  1 set of 15 rep warm-up
  sets of 10,8,8,8,8 reps
Lying Leg Curls: 5 sets + warm-up set
  1 set of 15 rep warm-up
  sets of 10,8,8,8,8 reps

Superset:
Standing Leg Curls: 5 sets
  10 reps each set
Straight-Leg Deadlifts: 5 sets
  10 reps each set

CALVES

Standing Calf Raises: 5 sets
  10 reps each set

Seated Calf Raises: 5 sets
  10 reps each set

ABDOMINALS

Bent-Knee Hanging Leg Raises: 100 reps
Crunches: 150 reps
Bent-Over Twists: 100 reps each side

CARDIOVASCULAR

Walk, Run, Bike, Swim, or Hike: 30-60 minutes

Tuesday / Thursday / Saturday

WARM-UP

Neck Rolls: 5 rolls to each side
Side Bends: 10 reps to each side
Lunges/Achilles Stretches: 5 combinations
Windmills: 20 reps to each side

ABDOMINALS

Roman Chair Sit-Ups: 5 minutes

SHOULDERS

Superset:
Behind-Neck Barbell Presses: 5 sets + warm-up set
  1 set of 15 rep warm-up
  sets of 10,8,8,8,6 reps
Dumbbell Lateral Raises: 5 sets
  8 reps each set

Superset:
Machine Front Press: 5 sets
   8 reps each set
Bent-Over Lateral Raises: 5 sets
   8 reps each set

Superset:
Upright Rows: 5 sets
   10 reps each set
One-Arm Seated Cable Laterals: 5 sets
   10 reps each set, each arm

UPPER ARMS

Superset:
Standing Barbell Curls: 5 sets
   sets of 15,10,8,6,6 reps
Lying French Presses: 5 sets
   sets of 15,10,8,6,6 reps

Superset:
Alternate Dumbbell Curls: 5 sets
   8 reps each set
Triceps Cable Pushdowns: 5 sets
   8 reps each set

Superset:
Concentration Curls: 5 sets
   8 reps each set
One-Arm Triceps Extensions: 5 sets
   12 reps each set
Reverse Push-Ups: 5 sets
   15 reps each set

FOREARMS

Superset:
Barbell Wrist Curls: 5 sets
  10 reps each set
Reverse Wrist Curls: 5 sets
  10 reps each set
One-Arm Wrist Curls: 5 sets
  10 reps each set

CALVES

Standing Calf Raises: 5 sets
  sets of 15,10,8,8,8 reps
Calf Raises On Leg Press Machine: 5 sets
  10 reps each set

ABDOMINALS

Bent-Knee Sit-Ups: 150 reps
Incline Board Leg Raises: 150 reps
Side Leg Raises: 100 reps each side
Hyperextensions: 3 set
  10 reps each set

CARDIOVASCULAR

Walk, Run, Bike, Swim, or Hike: 30-60 minutes

OVER 50 WORK-OUT (MEN & WOMEN)

Monday / Thursday

WARM-UP

Neck Rolls: 5 rolls to each side
Side Bends: 10 reps to each side
Lunges/Achilles Stretches: 5 combinations
Windmills: 20 reps to each side

CHEST

Barbell Bench Press: 3 sets + warm-up set
  1 set of 15 rep warm-up
  sets of 12,10,8 reps
Incline Barbell Bench Press: 3 sets
  sets of 12,10,8 reps
Dumbbell Flys: 3 sets
  sets of 12,10,8 reps
Dumbbell Pullovers: 3 sets
  12 reps each set

BACK

Lat Machine Pulldowns: 3 sets
  10 reps each set
Lat Machine Pulldowns - Close-Grip: 3 sets
  10 reps each set
Bent-Over Barbell Rows: 3 sets
  10 reps each set

THIGHS

Freehand Squats: 3 sets
  12 reps each set
Hack Squats: 3 sets
  sets of 12,10,8 reps
Lying Leg Curls: 3 sets
  sets of 15,12,10 reps
Standing Leg Curls: 3 sets
  10 reps each set

CALVES

Standing Calf Raises: 4 sets
  sets of 15,12,10,8 reps

ABDOMINALS

Bent-Over Twists: 50 reps each side
Crunches: 50 reps

CARDIOVASCULAR

Walk, Run, Bike, Swim, or Hike: 30-60 minutes

Tuesday / Friday

WARM-UP

Neck Rolls: 5 rolls to each side
Side Bends: 10 reps to each side
Lunges/Achilles Stretches: 5 combinations
Windmills: 20 reps to each side

SHOULDERS

Behind-Neck Barbell Presses: 3 sets + warm-up
  1 set of 15 rep warm-up
  sets of 12,10,8 reps
Dumbbell Lateral Raises: 3 sets
  12 reps each set
Dumbbell Shrugs: 3 sets
  10 reps each set

UPPER ARMS

Standing Barbell Curls: 3 sets
  sets of 15,12,10 reps
Concentration Curls: 3 sets
  10 reps each set
Triceps Cable Pushdowns: 3 sets
  10 reps each set

FOREARMS

Barbell Wrist Curls: 3 sets
  10 reps each set
Reverse Wrist Curls: 3 sets
  10 reps each set

CALVES

Seated Calf Raises: 4 sets
  sets of 15,12,10,8 reps

ABDOMINALS

Bent-Knee Sit-Ups: 50 reps
Incline Board Leg Raises: 50 reps

CARDIOVASCULAR

<u>Walk, Run, Bike, Swim, or Hike</u>: 30-60 minutes

Wednesday / Saturday

WARM-UP

<u>Neck Rolls</u>: 5 rolls to each side
<u>Side Bends</u>: 10 reps to each side
<u>Lunges/Achilles Stretches</u>: 5 combinations
<u>Windmills</u>: 20 reps to each side

ABDOMINALS

<u>Bent-Over Twists</u>: 50 reps each side
<u>Crunches</u>: 50 reps
<u>Bent-Knee Sit-Ups</u>: 50 reps
<u>Incline Board Leg Raises</u>: 50 reps

CARDIOVASCULAR

<u>Walk, Run, Bike, Swim, or Hike</u>: 60-90 minutes

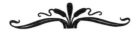

Definition of Terms and Proper Execution of Exercises

Aerobic Exercise: With oxygen. The muscles' demand for oxygen is met by the circulation of oxygen in the blood. Examples are: walking, swimming, long-distance running, etc.

Alternate Dumbbell Curls: Stand upright, a dumbbell in each hand hanging at arm's length. Curl one weight forward and up, holding your elbow steady at your waist and twisting your wrist slightly, bringing the thumb down and little finger up. Curl the weight as high as you can, then bring it back down under control through the same arc. Switch arms and repeat.

Anaerobic Exercise: Without oxygen. The oxygen demands of the muscles are so high that the circulatory system cannot supply adequate oxygen. Examples are: weight-lifting, sprinting, arm-wrestling, etc.

Barbell: A long bar with weights at both ends, designed to be used by both hands at once.

Barbell Bench Press: Lie on a flat bench, your feet on the floor for balance. Your grip should be wide enough so that as you lower the bar to your chest, your forearms should point straight up. Lift the bar off the rack and hold it at arm's length above you. Lower the bar slowly until it touches just below your pectoral muscles. The bar should come to a complete stop at this point. Press the bar upward until your arms are fully locked out.

Barbell Wrist Curls: Take hold of a barbell with an under-hand grip, hands close together. Straddle a bench with your forearms resting on the bench but with your wrists and hands hanging over the end, elbows and wrists the same distance apart. Lock your knees in against your elbows to stabilize them. Bend your wrists and lower the weight toward the floor. When you can't lower the bar any further, carefully open your fingers a little bit and let the weight roll down out of the palms of your hands. Roll the weight back into the palms of your hands, contract the forearms, and lift the weight as high as you can without letting your forearms come up off the bench.

Behind-Neck Barbell Presses: Sitting on a seated press bench, lift the barbell overhead (this is your starting position). Lower the bar behind your head slowly, letting the bar slightly touch your shoulders. Press the weight straight up to the starting position, keeping your elbows as far back as possible during the movement.

Bent-Knee Hanging Leg Raises: Take hold of a chin-up bar with an overhand grip and hang at arm's length from the bar. Bend your knees, then lift your legs as high as possible. Lower them back to the starting position. Do not swing while performing this exercise.

Bent-Knee Sit-Ups: Lie on your back, knees bent, feet flat on the floor, your hands on the outside of your thighs. Sit up and bring your head as close to your knees as possible. Lower yourself slowly back to the floor. Do this exercise slowly and always keep your chin pressed to your chest.

Bent-Over Lateral Raises: Sit on the end of a bench, knees together, and take a dumbbell in each hand. Bend forward from the waist and bring the dumbbells together behind your calves. Turn your hands so that your palms face one another. Keeping

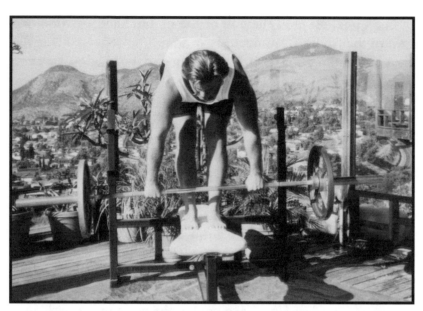

Bent-Over Barbell Rows: Standing with your feet a few inches apart, grasp the bar with a wide, overhand grip. With your knees slightly bent, bend forward until your upper body is about parallel to the floor. Keep your back straight and let the bar hang at arm's length below you, almost touching the shinbone. Lift the bar upward until it touches the upper abdominals, then slowly lower it again to the starting position.

your body steady, lift the weights out to either side, turning your wrists so that the thumbs are lower than the little fingers. With your arms slightly bent, lift the dumbbells to a point just higher than your head, then, keeping your knees together, lower them again slowly to a point behind your calves, resisting all the way down.

Bent-Over Twists: Stand upright, legs straight, feet shoulder width apart. Hold a broom handle across the back of your shoulders. Bend forward from the waist as far as comfortable. Turning from the waist but not letting the hips move at all, twist in one direction until the end of the broom handle is pointing toward the floor. Continue this windmill movement, swinging first in one direction, then back in the other direction.

Calf Raises on Leg Press Machine: Using a leg press machine, position yourself as if to do a leg press, only push against the foot pads with your toes, leaving your heels unsupported. Press the weight upward with your toes until fully extended, then let your toes come back toward you, feeling the fullest possible stretch in the calf muscles.

Cardiovascular Training: Cardiovascular training is an integral part of overall conditioning. These exercises strengthen the heart, lungs, and circulatory system. See *Aerobic Exercise*.

Close-Grip Chin-Ups: Take hold of the chin-up bar with your hands close together in an underhand grip. Pull yourself up, lean your head slightly back so that your chest nearly touches your hands. Lower your body back to the starting position.

Concentration Curls: In a standing position, bend over slightly and take a dumbbell in one hand. Rest your free arm on your knee to stabilize yourself. Curl the weight up to the deltoid without moving the upper arm or the elbow. Lower the weight slowly, resisting all the way down to full extension.

Crunches: Lie on your back on the floor. With your knees bent, raise your legs and place your feet against a wall or bench for support. Place your fingertips on your temples. Raise your head and shoulders toward your knees with a sit-up motion and simultaneously lift the pelvis and feel the contraction of the abdominals as the upper and lower body crunch together. Flex the abdominals to get the fullest possible contraction.

Donkey Calf Raises: Place your toes on a block, bend forward from the waist, and lean on a bench or table for support. Your toes should be directly below your hips. Have your training partner add resistance by seating her/himself across your hips, as far back as possible to keep pressure off the lower back. Lower your heels as far as possible, then come back up on your toes until your calves are fully contracted.

Dumbbell: A short bar with weights at both ends, intended for use with one hand at a time.

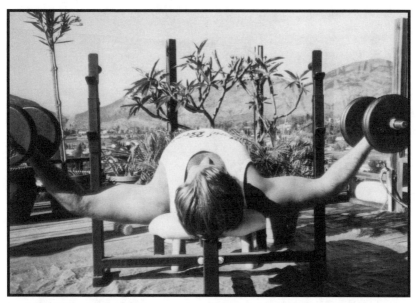

Dumbbell Flys: Lie on a bench holding dumbbells at arm's length above you, palms facing one another. Lower the weights out and down to either side in a wide arc as far as you can, feeling the pectoral muscles stretch to their maximum. The palms should remain facing each other throughout the movement. Bring the weights to a complete stop at a lower point than the bench, then lift them back up to the starting position along the same wide arc.

Dumbbell Incline Presses: Take a dumbbell in each hand and lie down on an incline bench. Lift the dumbbells to shoulder height, palms facing forward (this is your starting position). Press them simultaneously straight up overhead, then lower them back to the starting position. Vary the angle of the incline from workout to workout, or from set from set in the same workout.

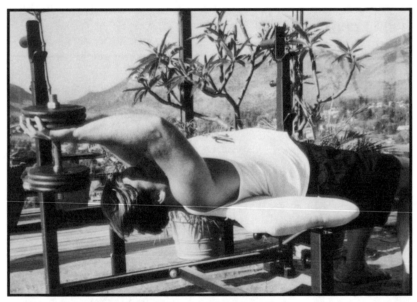

Dumbbell Pullovers: Lie across a bench with your feet flat on the floor. Place a dumbbell on the floor behind your head. Reach back and grasp the weight. Keeping your arms bent, raise the weight and bring it just over your head to your chest. Lower the weight slowly back to the starting position without touching the floor, feeling the lats stretch out to their fullest.

Dumbbell Lateral Raises: Take a dumbbell in each hand, bend forward slightly, and bring the weights together in front of you at arm's length. Lift the weights out and up to either side, turning your wrists slightly so the rear of the dumbbell is higher than the front. Lift the weights to a point slightly higher than your shoulders, then lower them slowly, resisting all the way down.

Dumbbell Shrugs: Stand upright, arms at sides, with a heavy dumbbell in each hand. Raise your shoulders as high as you can, as if trying to touch them to your ears. Hold at the top for a moment, then release and return to the starting position. Try not to move anything but your shoulders.

Freehand Squats: Stand straight up, flat-footed, arms crossed over your chest. Head up, back straight, feet 16 inches apart. Squat until upper thighs are parallel to floor. Return to starting position. Inhale down, exhale up.

Front Squats: Step up to the rack, bring your arms up under the bar, keeping the elbows high, cross your arms and grasp the bar with your hands to control it. Then lift the weight off the rack. Step back and separate your feet for balance. Bend your knees and, keeping your head up and your back straight, lower yourself until your thighs are below parallel to the floor. Push yourself back up to the starting position.

Hack Squats: Hook your shoulders under the padded bars. Your feet should be together, toes pointed slightly out. Press downward with your legs and lift the mechanism, stopping when your legs are fully extended. Bend your knees and lower yourself all the way down. Push yourself back up to the starting position.

Hyperextensions: Position yourself face down across a hyperextension bench, with your heels hooked under the rear supports. Clasp your hands across your chest or behind your head and bend forward and down as far as possible, feeling the lower back muscles stretch. From this position, come back up until your torso is just above parallel.

Incline Barbell Bench Press: Lie back on an incline bench. Reach up and grasp the bar with a medium-wide grip. Lift the bar off the rack and hold it straight overhead, arms locked. Lower the weight down to the upper chest, stop for a moment, then press it back up to the starting position.

Incline Board Leg Raises: Lie on your back on an incline board, head higher than your feet. Reach back and take hold of the top of the board or some other support. Keeping your legs straight and feet flexed, raise them up as high as you can, then lower them slowly, stopping just as they touch the board.

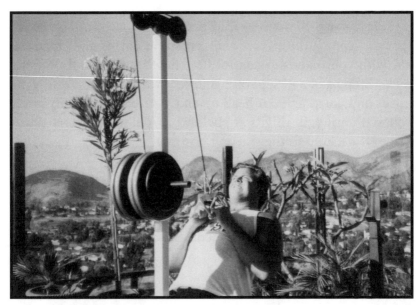

Lat Machine Pulldowns - Close Grip: Grasp the handles with a close grip with your knees hooked under the support. Pull the grip down smoothly until your hands slightly touch the top of your chest. Release, extend the arms again, and feel the lats fully stretch.

Breathing is very important while doing this exercise. As you raise your legs and compress the abdominal cavity, breathe out; as you lower your legs again, inhale deeply. Keep your chin tucked forward into the chest.

Incline Dumbbell Curls: Sit back on an incline bench holding a dumbbell in each hand. Keeping your elbows well forward throughout the movement, curl the weights forward and up to shoulder level. Lower the weights again, fully under control, and pause at the bottom to keep from swinging the weights up on the next repetition.

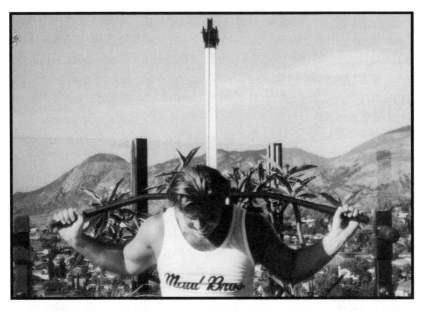

Lat Machine Pulldowns - Wide Grip: Using a long bar, grasp it with a wide, overhand grip with your knees hooked under the support. Pull the bar down smoothly until it touches the back of your neck, making the upper back do the work. Release, extend the arms again, and feel the lats fully stretch.

Lunges/Achilles Stretches: From a standing position with your feet together, step forward as far as you can with the left foot, keeping both feet pointed straight ahead. Bend your left knee and lower yourself as far as you can, keeping your back and your right leg straight. Put your hands down on either side of the forward foot for balance. Push up with your hands and straighten the left leg, but stay bent over with your hands remaining by your left foot. Keep both feet in place and flat on the floor, feeling the stretch in the back of your left leg and the Achilles' tendon of your right. Bend your head down as close as possible to the left knee. Slowly stand up and switch sides.

Lying Leg Curls: Lie face downward on a Leg Curl machine and hook your heels under the lever mechanism. Your legs should be stretched out straight. Keeping flat on the bench, curl your legs up as far as possible, until the leg biceps are fully contracted. Release and slowly lower the weight back to the starting position.

Lying Triceps Extensions: Lie along a bench, your head just off the end with knees bent and feet flat on the bench. Take hold of an E-Z bar with an overhand grip, hands about 10 inches apart. Press the weight up until your arms are locked out, but not straight up over your face (this is your starting position). Instead, the weight should be back behind the top of your head, with your triceps doing the work of holding it there. Keeping your elbows stationary, lower the weight down toward your forehead, then press it back up to the starting position, stopping just short of vertical.

Machine Front Press: Grasp the bar at shoulder level and press upward until your arms are locked out, then come back down slowly to the starting position, going through the longest range of motion possible.

Neck Rolls: Stand upright, hands at your sides. Breathe deeply, letting your shoulders, arms, and whole body relax as much as possible. Slowly rotate your head and neck to the left one complete circle. After one complete rotation to the left, do another one all the way around to the right.

One-Arm Seated Cable Laterals: Sitting on a stool or low bench, take hold of a handle attached to a floor-level pulley in such a way that your arm is fully extended across the front of your body. Keeping your body as still as possible, pull the handle across and up until your arm is fully extended to the side at about shoulder height. Lower the weight back to the starting position.

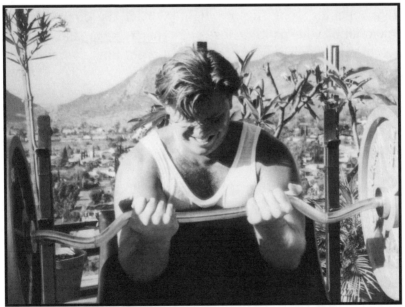

Preacher Curls: Position yourself with your chest against the bench, your arms extending over it. Take hold of an E-Z bar with an underhand grip. Curl the bar all the way up and then lower it again to full extension, resisting the weight on the way down. Flex the biceps at the top of the movement.

One-Arm Triceps Extensions: Sitting on a bench, take a dumbbell in one hand and hold it extended overhead. Keeping your elbow stationary and close to your head, lower the dumbbell down in an arc behind your head as far as you can. Feel the triceps stretch to their fullest, then press the weight back up to the starting position.

One-Arm Wrist Curls: Take hold of a dumbbell with one arm and sit on a bench. Lean forward and place your forearm on your thigh so that your wrist and the weight extend out over the knee, with your palm and the inside of your forearm facing upward. Bend forward, reach over with your free hand, and take hold of the elbow of the working arm to stabilize it. Bend your wrist and lower the weight as far as possible toward the floor, opening your fingers slightly to let the dumbbell roll down out of your palm. Close your fingers again and curl the weight up as high as you can. Finish repetitions, switch arms and repeat.

Parallel Dips: Taking hold of the parallel bars, raise yourself up and lock out your arms. As you bend your elbows and lower yourself between the bars, try to stay as upright as possible. From the bottom of the movement, press yourself back up until your arms are locked out, then flex pectorals and triceps to increase contraction.

Repetition (rep): One complete exercise movement, from starting position, through the full range of movement, then back to the beginning.

Reverse Push-Ups: Place a bench behind your back and hold onto the bench at its edge, hands about shoulder width apart. Place your heels on another bench at a level higher than the bench you are holding on to. Bending your elbows, lower your body as far as you can toward the floor. Then push back up, locking out your arms to work the upper triceps. Also known as "Bench Dips."

Reverse Wrist Curls: Grasp a barbell with an overhand grip, hands about 10 inches apart. Lay your forearms on top of your thighs so that they are parallel to the floor and your wrists and hands are free and unsupported. Bend your wrists forward and lower the bar as far as you can. Then bring them back up and lift the bar as far as possible, trying not to let the forearms move during the exercise.

Roman Chair Sit-Ups: Sit on the Roman Chair bench, hook your feet under the support, and fold your arms in front of you. Keeping your stomach tucked in, lower yourself to approximately a 70-degree angle. Raise yourself back up and come forward as far as possible, deliberately flexing and "crunching" your abdominal muscles to increase the contraction.

Seated Cable Rows: Take hold of the handles and sit with your feet braced against the crossbar, knees slightly bent. Extend your arms and bend forward slightly, feeling the lats stretch. From this beginning position, pull the handles back toward your body and touch them to your abdomen, feeling the back muscles doing most of the work. Your back should arch, your chest stick out, and try to touch the shoulder blades together as you draw the weight toward you. When the handles touch your abdomen you should be sitting upright. Keeping the weight under control, release and let the handles go forward again, once more stretching out the lats.

Seated Calf Raises: Sit on the machine and place your toes on the bottom crosspiece, hooking your knees under the crossbar. Slowly lower your heels as far toward the ground as possible, then press back up on your toes until your calves are fully contracted. Use a steady, rhythmic motion.

Set: A group of repetitions (reps). The number is arbitrary.
Programs designed to produce cardiovascular fitness generally
use high-repetition sets, while those that aim for strength use
fewer repetitions.

Side Bends: Stand upright, feet very wide apart. Raise your
right hand high overhead, and put your left hand down on the
side of your left leg. Stretch upward with your right arm as
high as you can, and then begin bending to your left, continu-
ing the stretch, and sliding your left hand down your left leg for
support. Hold for count of 5, then slowly return to starting position. Lower your right arm, raise your left, and repeat the Side
Bend to your right.

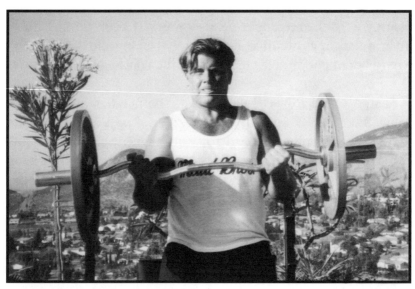

**Standing Curls: Stand with feet a few inches apart and
grasp an E-Z bar with an underhanded grip, hands about
shoulder width apart. Let the bar hang down at arm's
length in front of you. Curl the bar out and up in a wide
arc and bring it up as high as you can, your elbows close to
the body and stationary. Lower the weight, following the
same arc and resisting the weight all the way down until
your arms are fully extended.**

Side Leg Raises: Lie on your side supporting yourself on your elbow, your lower leg bent under for support. Keeping the upper leg straight, raise it slowly as high as it will go, then lower it again, but stopping short of letting it touch the floor. Don't move your hips at all during this movement.

Squats: With the barbell on a rack, step under it so that it rests across the back of your shoulders, hold on to the bar to balance it, raise up to lift it off the rack, and step away. Keeping your head up and your back straight, bend your knees and lower yourself until your thighs are just lower than parallel to the floor. From this point, push yourself back up to the starting position.

Standing Calf Raises: Stand with your toes on the block of a standing Calf Raise machine, your heels extended out into space. Hook your shoulders under the pads and straighten your legs, lifting the weight clear of the support. Lower your heels as far as possible toward the floor, keeping your knees slightly bent throughout the movement in order to work the lower area of the calves as well as the upper, and feeling the calf muscles stretch to the maximum. From the bottom of the movement, come up on your toes as far as possible.

Standing Leg Curls: Stand against the machine and hook one leg behind the lever mechanism. Hold yourself steady and curl the leg up as high as possible. Release and slowly lower the weight back to the starting position. Switch legs and repeat.

Straight-Leg Deadlifts: Place a barbell on the floor in front of you. Bend your knees, lean forward, and grasp the bar in a medium-wide grip, one hand in an overhand grip, the other in an underhand grip. Try to keep your back straight. Begin the lift by driving with your legs. Straighten up until you are standing upright, then throw the chest out and the shoulders back as

if coming to attention. Keep your legs locked and bend forward
from the waist, your back straight, until your torso is about parallel to the floor, the bar hanging at arm's length below you.
Straighten up again, pull your shoulders back, and arch your
back.

Stripping: The act of removing some weights from the bar at
the end of a set in order to squeeze out a few more reps that otherwise would not have been possible using the heavy weight
originally put on the bar.

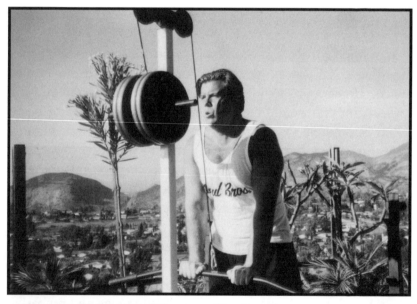

**Triceps Cable Pushdowns: Hook a bar to an overhead
cable and pulley, stand close to the bar and grasp it with an
overhand grip, hands about 10 inches apart. Keep your
elbows tucked in close to your body and stationary. Press
the bar down as far as possible, locking out your arms and
feeling the triceps contract fully. Release and let the bar
come up as far as possible without moving the elbows.**

Superset: A set of two or more exercises performed in a row without stopping (zero rest).

T-Bar Rows: Standing on a block with your feet close together, knees slightly bent, bend down and grasp the handles of the T-Bar machine with an overhand grip. Straighten your legs slightly and lift up until your body is at about a 45-degree angle. Without changing this angle, lift the weight up until it touches your chest, then lower it again to arm's length, keeping the weight off the floor.

Upright Rows: Stand grasping a barbell with an overhand grip, hands a few inches apart. Let the bar hang down in front of you. Lift it straight up, keeping it close to your body, until the bar just about touches your chin. From the top, lower it once more under control to the starting position.

Wide-Grip Chin-Ups: Take hold of the chin-up bar with an overhand grip, hands as wide apart as practicable. Hang from the bar, then pull yourself up so that the back of your neck touches the bar. Hold for a brief moment, then lower yourself slowly back to the starting position.

Windmills: Stay in the bent-over position, straighten your arms out to each side, and twist so that you touch your right hand to your left foot. Your left arm should remain straight and end up pointing at the sky. At the same time, turn your head so that you are looking up behind you. Repeat the movement to the other side, touching your left hand to your right foot.

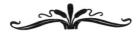

Seasonal Produce Availability

The seasonal availability of fruits and vegetables is Nature's way of telling you what to eat and when. Eating foods when they are in season is an integral part of health and the importance of doing so cannot be overemphasized. Thus, I have included the following information regarding seasonal produce availability. Though varieties of each food may differ, this compilation lists each food's peak season(s) according to a survey of Farmer's Markets conducted within the United States in 2002.

Compiled by Stephen and Jolie Arlin

Food	**Season**
Acorn Squash	Summer
Almond	Fall
Ambrosia Melon	Summer
Anise	Fall
Apple	Fall, Early Winter
Apricot	Summer
Arrame	All seasons
Artichoke	Fall
Arugula	Winter
Asian Pear	Fall, Early Winter
Asparagus	Spring
Atemoya	Late Winter, Spring
Avocado	All seasons
Banana	All seasons
Basil	All seasons
Beet	Fall, Winter, Spring

Food	Season
Blackberry	Early Summer
Black Sapote	Summer
Blood Orange	Winter
Blueberry	Summer
Bok Choy	Winter
Boysenberry	Early Summer
Brazil Nut	Fall
Breadfruit	Early Summer
Broccoli	Winter
Brussels Sprouts	Fall
Cabbage	Winter
Canistel	Spring
Cantaloupe	Summer
Carambola	Spring
Carob	Spring
Carrot	All seasons
Casaba Melon	Summer
Cashew Apple	Fall
Cassia	Spring
Cauliflower	Winter
Celery	Fall
Chard	Fall, Winter, Spring
Chayote	Fall
Cherimoya	Late Winter, Spring
Cherry	Spring
Chestnut	Fall
Chicory	Fall, Winter, Spring
Chive	All seasons
Cilantro	All seasons
Cranberry	Fall
Crenshaw Melon	Summer
Coconut	All seasons
Collard	Fall, Winter, Spring

Food	Season
Corn	Summer
Currant	Spring
Cucumber	Summer
Dandelion	Late Winter, Spring
Date	Fall, Winter
Dill	All seasons
Dulse	All seasons
Durian	Spring, Summer
Eggplant	Summer
Endive	Fall
Escarole	Fall, Winter, Spring
Fennel	Winter
Feijoa	Fall
Fiddlehead Fern	Fall, Winter, Spring
Fig	Late Summer
Frisee	Fall, Winter, Spring
Garlic	All seasons
Ginger	All seasons
Ginseng	All seasons
Gooseberry	Summer
Gourd	Fall
Grapefruit	Winter, Early Spring
Grape	Summer
Green Bean	Early Summer
Green Butter	Fall, Winter, Spring
Green Leaf	Fall, Winter, Spring
Green Oak	Fall, Winter, Spring
Guava	Spring
Hazelnut	Fall
Hijiki	All seasons
Honeydew Melon	Summer
Huckleberry	Late Summer
Jakfruit	Spring

Food	Season
Jicama	All seasons
Jujube	Fall
Kale	Fall, Winter, Spring
Kiwi	Winter, Early Spring
Kohlrabi	Fall, Winter, Spring
Kombu	All seasons
Kumquat	Winter
Lamb's Quarters	Winter
Leeks	Fall
Lemonberry	Summer
Lemongrass	Winter
Lemon	Winter, Early Spring
Lime	Winter, Early Spring
Loganberry	Early Summer
Longan	Summer
Loquat	Early Summer
Lotus	All seasons
Lovage	Spring, Summer
Lychee	Summer
Macadamia Nut	Fall
Mache	Fall, Winter, Spring
Malva	Late Fall, Winter
Mamey Sapote	Spring
Mango	Late Spring, Summer
Mangosteen	Fall, Early Summer
Marjoram	All seasons
Mint	All seasons
Mizuna	Fall, Winter, Spring
Monstera Deliciosia	Late Spring, Summer
Mountain Apple	Spring
Mulberry	Summer
Mustard	Fall, Winter, Spring
Nasturtium	Summer

Food	Season
Nectarine	Summer
Nori	All seasons
Okra	Fall
Olive	Fall, Winter, Spring
Onion	All seasons
Orange	Winter, Early Spring
Oregano	All seasons
Papaya	All seasons
Parsley	All seasons
Parsnip	Late Fall
Passionfruit	Fall
Peach	Summer
Peanut	All seasons
Pear	Fall, Early Winter
Pea	Spring
Pecan	Fall
Pepper	Late Summer, Fall
Peppergrass	All seasons
Persimmon	Fall
Pineapple	All seasons
Pine Nut	Fall
Pistachio	Fall
Plantain	All seasons
Plum	Early Summer
Pomegranate	Fall
Pomelo	Winter
Potato	All seasons
Prickly Pear	Fall
Pumpkin	Fall
Purslane	All seasons
Quince	Fall, Early Winter
Radicchio	Fall, Winter, Spring
Radish	Fall, Winter

Food	**Season**
Rambutan	Summer
Raspberry	Early Summer
Red Butter	Fall, Winter, Spring
Red Chard	Fall, Winter, Spring
Red Oak	Fall, Winter, Spring
Red Orach	Fall, Winter, Spring
Rhubarb	Spring
Rosemary	All seasons
Rutabaga	Late Fall
Sage	All seasons
Sapodilla	Spring
Savory	Fall, Winter, Spring
Scallion	All seasons
Sea Palm	All seasons
Shallot	All seasons
Sharlyn Melon	Summer
Snow Pea	Early Spring
Sorrel	Late Winter
Sourgrass	All seasons
Soursop	Late Winter, Spring
Spinach	Winter
Strawberry	Summer
Sugar Apple	Late Winter, Spring
Summer Squash	Summer
Sunflower	Summer
Surinam Cherry	Spring
Sweet Potato	Fall
Tamarind	Spring
Tangelo	Winter, Early Spring
Tangerine	Winter, Early Spring
Tango	Fall, Winter, Spring
Tarragon	All seasons
Tat Soi	Fall, Winter, Spring

Food	Season
Thyme	All seasons
Tiger Lily	Summer
Tomatillo	Late Summer
Tomato	Summer
Travissio	Fall, Winter, Spring
Turnip	Winter
Ugli Fruit	Winter, Early Spring
Velvet Apple	Late Summer
Violet	Summer
Wakame	All seasons
Walnut	Fall
Watercress	Fall, Winter, Spring
Watermelon	Summer
Wheatgrass	All seasons
White Sapote	Winter, Summer
Wintercress	All seasons
Winter Squash	Fall, Winter
Yam	Fall
Zucchini	Early Summer

There are many thousands more edible foods in the world. You could eat a different raw plant food every day of your life and *still* not try them all! Does anyone still think that eating a raw-food diet is boring?

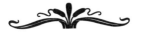

Conclusions

*To go places you have not gone,
you have to do things you have not done.*

Maintain your emotional poise. Release worry, fear, anxiety, jealousy, stress, nervousness, and neurosis through physical movement of the body, through the free flow of body energy, and through deep breathing. Take your aggressions out by engaging in anaerobic exercise.

Boxers, horse trainers, and successful athletes have long understood that abstinence from sex before a competition maintains strength. Overindulgence in sex with the resultant loss of nutrients during ejaculation, causes weight loss and energy depletion. After ejaculation, nutrients designed for other vital organs, are sidetracked into the production of reproductive materials. This depletion results in a momentary insufficiency in the nutrients available to other biological systems of the body. Sex is wonderful, but engage in sex at the appropriate times—not before a work-out or contest!

Be true. The only fools are those who fool themselves. I have a quote in my book **Nature's First Law: The Raw-Food Diet** you should keep in mind: "The idea that natural nutrition may be followed by unnatural and harmful effects is an absurd notion which should be abandoned once and for all." Nutrition is no science—it is very simple. Live by the Laws of Nature and you shall prosper; live by the laws of civilization and you shall perish. All weight loss and emaciation due to The Raw-Food Diet is a result of the "good pushing out the bad" and other catabolic detoxification processes. The strength and weight will build if one is persistent.

The major problem that is plaguing humanity is addiction. Addiction to toxicity; addiction to being in a toxic physiological condition actually. People are constantly trying to reach a level of euphoria artificially, which is theirs naturally. When you are 100% raw for an extended period of time, it is a magical experience. Again, there is no magic pill, but there is a magic process to achieving perfect health. If people would just adhere to, and trust in, the Laws of Nature, they could begin to realize their true potential, their life's true meaning on this planet. Try it for yourself...and you shall be convinced.

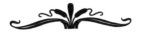

Recommended Reading

A Raw-Food Doctor's Cure, Dr. O.L.M. Abramowski
Biological Transmutations, Louis Kervran
Blatant Raw-Foodist Propaganda, Joe Alexander
Children of the Sun, Gordon Kennedy
The Children's Health Food Book, Ron Seaborn
Colon Health: The Key to a Vibrant Life, Dr. Norman Walker
The Complete Book of Juicing, Michael Murray
Confessions of a Medical Heretic, Dr. Robert Mendelsohn
Conscious Eating, Dr. Gabriel Cousens
Die Sonnen-Diat: Ein vegetarisches Programm fur Vitalitat und Superfitness (German), David Wolfe
Diet for a New America, John Robbins
Dr. Jensen's Guide to Better Bowel Care, Bernard Jensen
Eating for Beauty, David Wolfe
Edible Wild Plants, Elias & Dykeman
Enzyme Nutrition, Dr. Edward Howell
Fast Food Nation: The Dark Side of the All American Meal, Eric Schlosser
Feel-Good Food: A Guide to Intuitive Eating, Susie Miller & Karen Knowler
Food Combining & Digestion, Steve Meyerowitz
Food Enzymes, Humbart Santillo
Fountain of Youth, Arnold DeVries
Fresh Vegetable and Fruit Juices, Dr. Norman Walker
Fruit: Best of All Foods, Klaus Wolfram
Fruit: The Food and Medicine for Man, Morris Krok
Garden of Eden Raw Fruit and Vegetable Recipes, Phyllis Avery
Gardening Without Digging, A. Guest

The Healing Miracles of Coconut Oil, Bruce Fife
Hippocrates Diet & Health Program, Ann Wigmore
Hooked on Raw, Rhio
Introducing Living Foods to Your Child: Guidebook for Babies through Two Years, Beth Montgomery
Inventing The AIDS Virus, Dr. Peter Duesberg
IS Philosophy, Stephen Arlin
It's All in Your Head, Dr. Hal Huggins
Juice Fasting and Detoxification, Steve Meyerowitz
The Juicing Book, Stephen Blauer
Juicing for Life, Cherie Calbom and Maureen Keane
The Juiceman's Power of Juicing, Jay Kordich
Lick the Sugar Habit, Nancy Appleton
Living Foods for Optimum Health, Brian Clement
The Living Foods Lifestyle, Brenda Cobb
Living in the Raw, Rose Lee Calabro
Mad Cowboy, Howard Lyman
Major Achievements of the Cooked-Food Eater, Stephen Arlin
Man's Higher Consciousness, Hilton Hotema
Meditation: The First and Last Freedom, Osho
Mucusless Diet Healing System, Arnold Ehret
Naked Empress: The Great Medical Fraud, Hans Ruesch
Nature's First Law: The Raw-Food Diet, Stephen Arlin, Fouad Dini, David Wolfe
On Form and Actuality, David Wolfe
Our Precious Pets, Ann Wigmore
Overcoming AIDS & Other Incurable Diseases, Ann Wigmore
Physical Fitness through a Superior Diet, Arnold Ehret
Primal Mothering in a Modern World, Hygeia Halfmoon
Power Juices Super Drinks, Steve Meyerowitz
Prostate Enlarged? Try Nature's Way, Joe Daigre
Rational Fasting, Professor Arnold Ehret
Raw: The Uncook Book, Juliano

Raw Courage World, R.C. Dini
Raw Family, The Boutenko Family
The Raw Gourmet, Nomi Shannon
Raw Kids, Cheryl Stoycoff
Raw Knowledge, Paul Nison
The Raw Life, Paul Nison
The Raw Truth: The Art of Loving Foods, Jeremy Safron
    & Renee Underkoffler
Recipes for Longer Life, Ann Wigmore
Rohkost statt Feuerkost (German), Helmut Wandmaker
Secrets to Optimal Natural Breathing, Mike White
Shazzie's Detox Delights, Shazzie
Spiritual Nutrition and The Rainbow Diet, Dr. Gabriel
    Cousens
Spiritualizing Dietetics: Vitarianism, Johnny Lovewisdom
Sprouts: the Miracle Food, Steve Meyerowitz
The Sunfood Diet Success System, David Wolfe
Sunfood Cuisine, Frederic Patenaude
Sunlight, Dr. Zane Kime
Superior Nutrition, Herbert Shelton
Survival in the 21st Century, Viktoras Kulvinskas
The Teenage Liberation Handbook, Grace Llewellyn
Think Before You Eat, Diane Olive
Thus Speaketh the Stomach, Arnold Ehret
**Twelve Steps to Raw Foods: How to End Your Addiction
    to Cooked Food**, Victoria Boutenko
UnCooking with Jamey & Kim, Jameth Dina & Kim Sproul
The Unschooling Handbook, Mary Griffith
Viva's Healthy Dining Guide, Lisa Margolin & Connie Dee
Wheatgrass: Nature's Finest Medicine, Steve Meyerowitz
The Wheatgrass Book, Ann Wigmore
Willst Du gesund sein? Vergiß den Kochtopf! (German),
    Helmut Wandmaker
Whole Foods Companion, Diane Onstad
Yoga Gave Me Superior Health, Theos Bernard

The Yoga Tradition, George Feuerstein
Your Body's Many Cries For Water, Dr. Batmanghelidj MD

Also Recommended:
How to Win an Argument with a Cooked-Food Eater
   (audio tape), Stephen Arlin
Nature's First Law Videos, CD's, & Audio Tapes
Sunfire Cuisine (video)
Raw Yoga (video)
Just Eat An Apple Magazine
FRESH Network News

All books, magazines, and tapes available through:
Nature's First Law
PO Box 900202
San Diego, CA 92190 USA
(800) 205-2350
(619) 596-7979
(619) 645-7282
(619) 596-7997 (fax)
Internet: http://www.rawfood.com
Email: nature@rawfood.com

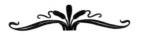

Resources

Stephen Arlin & David Wolfe
Nature's First Law
The world's premier source of raw-food diet books, juicers,
raw/organic food, superfoods, videos, tapes, retreats, etc.
PO Box 900202
San Diego, CA 92190 USA
619-645-7282
800-205-2350
888-RAW-FOOD
Internet: http://www.rawfood.com
E-mail: nature@rawfood.com

Creative Health Institute (CHI)
Health educators in Michigan.
918 Union City Rd.
Union City, MI 49094
517-278-6260

FRESH Network News
Raw-food magazine that promotes
The Raw-Food Diet in the UK and abroad.
To subscribe, contact:
Nature's First Law
619-645-7282
www.rawfood.com

Hippocrates Health Institute
Health resort in Florida.
1443 Palmdale Court
West Palm Beach, FL 33411
800-842-2125

Just Eat An Apple Magazine
From the Nature's First Law head office: This is the world's premier magazine on The Raw-Food Diet.
To subscribe, contact:
Nature's First Law
619-645-7282
www.rawfood.com

Karyn's Fresh Corner
Raw-food restaurant in Chicago.
3351 North Lincoln Ave.
Chicago, IL 60657
773-296-6990

Living Community Center
Raw resource center in Arizona.
330 East Seventh Street
Tucson, Arizona
520-623-0913

Living Light Culinary Arts Institute
Living-foods preparation classes.
704 N. Harrison
Fort Bragg, CA 95437
800-484-6933, ext. 6256

Living Light House
Hosts raw-food events in Southern California.
1457 12th Street
Santa Monica, CA 90401
310-395-6337

Nature's First Law Raw Superstore
Source for everything RAW!
1567 N. Cuyamaca St.
El Cajon, CA 92020
(800) 205-2350
(619) 596-7979
http://www.rawfood.com

Optimum Health Institute
Raw-food healing center in San Diego.
6970 Central Ave.
Lemon Grove, CA 91945
619-464-3346

Quintessence
Raw-food restaurant in New York City.
263 East 10th Street
New York City, NY 10009
(located between 1st Ave. and Avenue A)
646-654-1823

Raw Foods Foundation
Raw foods group in the St. Louis area.
HC 77, Box 41
Annapolis, MO 63620
314-725-6085

The Raw Truth Cafe, Healing Center, And Eco-Shop
Raw-food restaurant in Las Vegas.
3620 East Flamingo Road
Las Vegas, NV 89121
702-450-9007

Rhio's Raw Energy Hotline
Raw-Food Diet support in New York.
212-343-1152

San Diego County Living Foods Group
Raw foods group in San Diego.
P.O. Box 3397
Vista, CA 92085-3397
619-360-6968

Barbara Simonsohn
Germany's premier raw-foodist.
Holbeinstr. 26
27607 Hamburg
Germany
+ 49 (0) 40 895 338

Super Sprouts
Raw resource center in Toronto.
205 Spadina Ave.
Toronto, Ontario
M5T 2C8
Canada
416-977-7796

Tree of Life Rejuvenation Center
Healing retreat center headed by Dr. Cousens.
P.O. Box 1080
Patagonia, AZ 85624
520-394-2520

Wandmaker Aktuell
A German raw-food magazine.
Helmut-Wandmaker-Stiftung
Hauptstrasse 4, D-25782 Tellingstedt
Germany
04838-78047

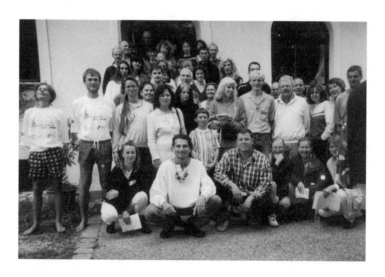

**David Wolfe and Stephen Arlin (front row)
team up with Germany's premier raw-foodist,
Barbara Simonsohn (2nd row, long blond hair),
for a weekend retreat in Munich, Germany.**

Visit our Raw-Food Superstore and Office, located at:
Nature's First Law
1567 North Cuyamaca St.
El Cajon, CA 92020 U.S.A.
(near San Diego, California)

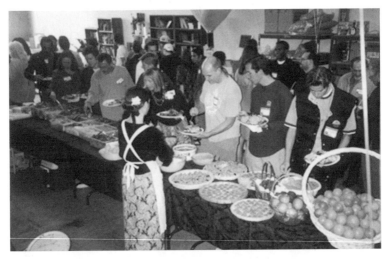

A spectacular array of raw gourmet dishes served at one
of our lecture/luncheons. Jolie's food is amazing!

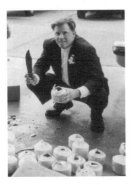 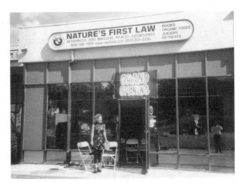

Call for directions and/or event reservations:
(619) 596-7979 or (800) 205-2350
Online maps: http://www.rawfood.com/directions.html
Open to the public Monday-Friday, 10:00am to 4:00pm
Raw/organic foods, books, 21st century appliances, etc.

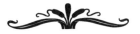

Contact Us!

If you have any questions or comments about any of the material contained in this book, feel free to contact Stephen Arlin and Nature's First Law. To receive free e-mail bulletins (concerning upcoming events, new products, monthly specials, exciting news, media coverage, etc.) from Nature's First Law and Stephen Arlin, send an e-mail to: nature@rawfood.com requesting to be added to the subscriber list.

Additional copies of **Raw Power!** may be ordered directly from Nature's First Law. One book is $14.95 plus $4.50 for Priority shipping and handling ($10.00 s&h if outside the United States or Canada). For each additional book please add $2.00 shipping (add $6.50 s&h if outside the United States or Canada). California residents add 7.75% sales tax. **Bulk discounts are available.**

Also, check out the **Nature's First Law Catalog**. The catalog contains many popular, rare, and exotic books, juicers, raw/organic food, videos, audios, etc. on The Raw-Food Diet. To receive a free copy of the Nature's First Law Catalog please write, call, or e-mail Nature's First Law.

Stephen Arlin
Nature's First Law
PO Box 900202
San Diego, CA 92190 U.S.A.
(619) 645-7282 / (800) 205-2350 - orders only
E-mail: nature@rawfood.com
Internet Homepage: http://www.rawfood.com

Our aspirations are our possibilities.